HIIT: How to Lose Weight, Get Shredded Muscles and Improve Your Health with High-Intensity Interval Training

by Mark Jones

Disclaimer:

This book is for informational purposes only. The publisher and author of this book are not responsible in any manner whatsoever for any damages arising directly or indirectly from use of the information in this book.

None of the claims in this book should be construed as medical advice. Consult with a medical professional prior to making any changes in your life that could impact your health.

High-intensity interval training carries a higher risk of injury and bodily harm than normal exercise because of the stress and strain it puts on the body of those who participate in it. Use the information in this book at your own risk. The publisher and author disclaim any liabilities for damages caused by use of the information contained herein.

Contents

What Is HIIT?

Just a few short years ago, exercise physiologists believed cardio exercises that raised the heart rate and kept it steady at a moderate rate throughout an entire cardio session was the best form of aerobic exercise for losing weight. They believed that lower-intensity exercise was more effective than high-intensity exercise because the body burned more fat for fuel during extended low-intensity sessions.

As it turns out, they couldn't have been more wrong. HIIT flips that theory on its head, instead opting to have you go all out for brief periods of time, followed by intervals of light to moderate difficulty between the intense sessions.

HIIT is an acronym for **High-Intensity Interval Training**. This relative newcomer to the world of fitness is a form of exercise in which intense sessions of anaerobic exercise are combined with recovery periods consisting of low-intensity exercises to create a training session that is believed to be superior to traditional steady-state aerobic training sessions when it comes to burning fat and building muscle. Additionally, HIIT has been shown to increase cardiovascular ability, improve cholesterol and lower insulin sensitivity.

An example of a simple HIIT session would be 20 minutes worth of intervals of sprinting at full speed for 30 seconds, followed by light jogging for 60 seconds. The 30-second interval is the **high-intensity interval**. It may not seem like much, but is kept short by design, so the exerciser is able to sustain maximum exertion. The 60 seconds of light cardio makes up what is known as the **active recovery interval**, which is time spent engaging in light exercise between the high-intensity intervals in order to allow your body to recharge a bit before the next high-intensity interval begins.

HIIT workouts tend to be shorter than regular workouts, with some of the shortest HIIT workouts clocking in at less than 5 minutes. Don't assume a shorter workout is going to be easier, as newcomers to HIIT often find themselves drenched in sweat and sucking for breath. High-intensity interval training sessions are compact, but there's mounting evidence that appears to prove they're a better choice than steady-state cardio.

While the typical cardio session often ends up feeling like a drawn-out torture session, HIIT offers a more compact workout with sessions of active recovery mixed in. HIIT sessions aren't easy, but a number of exercisers, amateur and professional alike, have found the shorter sessions to be more tolerable than longer cardio sessions.

While most new trends in the world of exercise prove to be nothing more than passing fads, it appears that HIIT is here to stay. HIIT sessions can be designed to fit your individual needs and will produce the results you're looking for quickly. What more could you ask for from a training session?

HIIT Training vs. Interval Training

All high-intensity interval training involves intervals, but not all interval training qualifies as HIIT. There are a lot of people who are engaging in interval training and are calling it HIIT, but aren't actually doing HIIT. I hear guys at the gym all the time claiming to be doing hour-long HIIT routines. When I watch what they're doing, I find they're doing interval training, but it falls short of being actual HIIT.

Interval training involves switching back and forth between different intensities of intervals in a single training session. HIIT does the same thing, but steps it up to the next level by switching between full-intensity intervals and moderate-intensity intervals. If you aren't giving 100% of what you're capable of on every high-intensity interval, you aren't doing HIIT.

Most exercisers aren't capable of giving everything they've got for more than about 30 seconds. A minute of maximum-intensity effort will drain all but the most elite of athletes. The active recovery periods are designed to allow the exerciser just enough time to recover from the maximum-intensity interval to do it again.

Interval training is effective in its own right, but HIIT seeks to step intervals up to a whole new level. HIIT workouts are short by design, usually clocking in at less than 30 minutes (including warm-up and cool-down periods), because most people aren't able to sustain the high level of effort required during HIIT intervals for more than about 20 minutes. If you are able to make it past the 30-minute mark with your intervals, it's probably because you aren't giving it everything you have during the high-intensity interval portions of your routine.

Remember this when determining whether your workout qualifies as a HIIT routine. If you've still got anything left in the gas tank at the end of the workout, it probably wasn't HIIT. High-intensity interval training demands that you put it all on the line. If you still have something left to give, you may not have HIIT it hard enough.

The Many Benefits of HIIT

In addition to weight loss, the following health benefits are believed to be attributed to HIIT:

- **Boosted metabolism.**
- **Effective fat burning.**
- **Endurance gains.**
- **Improved insulin resistance.**
- **Improvements in cardiovascular health.**
- **Improvements in oxygen uptake.**
- **Reduced muscle loss.**
- **Lower blood pressure.**

As you can see, there are a number of benefits associated with HIIT. It's considered one of the best ways to torch fat and it does so in a compact workout that takes up 30 minutes of your day or less.

The Science behind HIIT

While HIIT is currently trending in the world of fitness, there's a decent amount of scientific evidence that appears to back up the claim that shorter bursts of intense exercise are superior to longer sessions of moderate cardio. A number of recent studies have produced results that show HIIT to be an effective means of losing weight, trimming inches off the waistline and improving overall health.

A study published in the Metabolism journal in 1994 compared the effect of both HIIT and endurance training on body fat and skeletal muscle metabolism in healthy young adults. The participants in the study were subjected to either a 15-week HIIT program or a longer 20-week endurance training program. The estimated energy expended by participants in the endurance training program was roughly double that of the participants in the HIIT program, but they didn't see anywhere near double the results. In fact, when adjusted to account for the difference in energy expenditure, the participants in the HIIT program lost more than triple the body fat than those in the steady-state exercise group (1).

Sprint interval training (SIT), which will be covered in-depth in a later chapter, is a form of HIIT in which full-speed sprints are combined with either rest or active recovery periods.

A 2010 study looked at the effect of SIT training on overweight and obese men and found that participants who completed a 2-week SIT intervention consisting of 30-

second sprints followed by 4 ½ minute rest periods showed a significant reduction in both waist and hip circumference. Oxygen uptake and insulin sensitivity showed marked improvement after sprint interval training and systolic blood pressure was lower for at least 24 hours post-intervention. This effect was short-lived, as blood pressure, insulin sensitivity and oxygen uptake all returned to close to baseline when measurements were taken 72 hours after the intervention (2).

What this appears to indicate is HIIT exercise can help you lose inches off both your waistline and your hips, with the added bonus of potentially lowering blood pressure and improving insulin sensitivity. HIIT may even help you breathe easier and more deeply, but the effects are going to be short-lived if you stop exercising and return to leading a sedentary lifestyle.

A 2005 study looked at the connection between intensity of exercise and its effect on blood lipids. The participants were asked to perform 8 different exercises consisting of 20 repetitions of a light load or 8 exercises of 10 repetitions of a heavier load. They were then asked to wait 7 days, after which they were asked to perform whichever of the sets of exercises they hadn't previously performed. Blood was drawn before, right after and 15 minutes after the last exercise was complete. It was determined that intense exercise increased HDL cholesterol, which is good cholesterol in the body, immediately after high-intensity exercise (3).

These are just a handful of the many studies that seem to indicate HIIT is more than just a passing fad. Here are a few more that appear to tie HIIT to a number of health benefits:

- A 2008 University of South Wales study of the effect of HIIT on young women found performing HIIT 3 times a week for 15 weeks produced significant reductions in total body fat while improving insulin resistance when compared to the same amount of steady-state exercise (4).
- A study of subjects who cycle regularly found that aerobic power, exercise work rates and peak power output were all increased after interval training (5).
- An East Tennessee State University study of obese women found that HIIT improved aerobic power, body composition and resting metabolic rate when compared to low-intensity steady state training (6).

Most of the studies of HIIT have been published in the last 10 years and have produced largely positive results. HIIT appears to be an effective means of lowering body fat while taking inches off of all of the areas that matter. It also appears to be a means through which you can maximize weight loss while minimizing the amount of muscle being lost to atrophy.

Keep a watchful eye on the studies of HIIT currently being done by the scientific community. Since HIIT is a relative newcomer to the world of fitness, it's highly likely that all of the health benefits haven't yet been discovered.

There may be additional health benefits of HIIT just waiting to be unlocked.

Marathon Runners vs. Sprinters

In case you need further proof HIIT allows you to lose fat while retaining and possibly even building muscle, let's take a quick look at the difference between marathon runners and Olympic sprinters.

At a glance, you'll immediately notice marathon runners are thin and appear to have little by way of muscle on their bodies. These runners endure long, intense training sessions designed to improve their stamina to the point where they're able to run long distances while maintaining a certain speed. Marathon runners don't run fast. Instead, they run for a long time at a slower speed than the top speed they're capable of. Elite marathon athletes often find themselves running in excess of 100 miles per week, placing them firmly at the extreme end of steady-state athletes.

Extended periods of aerobic exercise isn't conducive to muscle growth, so marathon runners tend to be thin and lanky. To be fair, Olympic marathon runners are in prime condition and are elite athletes who are able to withstand rigorous training regimens; they just don't tend to have much muscle mass on their bodies.

On the other hand, an Olympic sprinter is more often than not a sight to behold. Olympic sprinters have bulging muscles and have significantly more muscle mass than marathon runners. Sprinters train every bit as hard as marathon runners, but they don't train for endurance. They train for short bursts of intense speed because they aren't in their races for the long haul. They're looking to win a short race run at the fastest speeds humanly possible. In short, they fall at the extreme end of high-intensity training.

While nobody would make the argument that marathon runners are out of shape, I would argue that I'd rather look like a sprinter than a marathon runner when it's all said and done. Not that looking like a marathon runner is a bad thing; I'd just rather have all my hard work pay off in added muscle mass combined with fat loss instead of fat loss at the expense of muscle mass.

Short, fast bursts of intense cardio exercise will help you to lose fat without robbing your body of muscle size and fullness. If there's any doubt, look up pictures of marathon runners and sprinters on your computer and compare them side-by-side.

HIIT Burns More Calories

The intensity and duration of HIIT intervals allows you to really step up the pace of your workout, which results in your body burning a larger number of calories in a shorter amount of time. A good HIIT routine can burn more calories in 20 minutes of work than most people burn in an hour of steady-state cardio.

The real benefit of HIIT lies in something known amongst HIIT enthusiasts as the **"afterburn."** This is the effect HIIT has on the body after the workout, as the body continues to burn calories well after the workout is complete in an attempt to restore itself back to a resting state. This afterburn effect is believed to last for a day or two after an intense HIIT workout. This effect is practically non-existent when it comes to steady-state cardio.

It's recommended you space your HIIT workouts out with a day or two between them in order to take full advantage of afterburn effect. Your body hasn't fully recovered a day later and you'll be placing additional stress on it by working out too soon.

Why Are HIIT Routines So Short?

When it comes to cardio, people are under the impression that longer sessions of moderate-speed cardio are the way to go when it comes to burning calories and eliminating fat. This is largely because that's the way it's been taught for decades. These people scoff at the idea of a 20- to 30-minute HIIT session because they feel 60 minutes on the treadmill at a low incline and moderate speed is the way to go.

HIIT workouts are short by design because you're expected to leave it all on the line during the high-intensity portions of intervals. Giving it all you've got during multiple intervals during a HIIT session should exhaust you to the point where you wouldn't be able to do more than a 20- to 30-minute session. HIIT should be exhausting for amateurs and veterans alike, because regardless of skill level, the exerciser is supposed to put everything he or she has into the intense intervals.

The short active recovery periods aren't anywhere near enough to fully recover. They're designed to give you a breather, so you can build up enough energy to go hard again when the next interval starts. By the time a HIIT session ends, you should be short of breath and dripping sweat, with little left in the reserves.

If you're doing HIIT right and are getting your heart rate and exhaustion level into the right zones during your intervals, you'll leave the gym feeling more tired after a

HIIT session than you would if you'd done 60 minutes of steady-state cardio.

While the HIIT workout itself won't burn a ton of calories, the afterburn effect mentioned previously coupled with the calories burnt during the workout will result in more calories burnt and increased fat loss in comparison to steady-state workouts that take much longer.

HIIT routines are short because they need to be short in order to ensure the exerciser can push hard during the high-intensity intervals without having to worry about burning out before the routine is complete. They're short by design, and are highly effective *because* of their length.

You'll realize the same benefits and then some when comparing HIIT to longer steady-state cardio routines. It isn't the length of the workout that matters inasmuch as it's the effort put into it.

Getting Ready for HIIT

If you hop on the Internet and search for HIIT workouts with the intent of doing the first workout you find, you may be in for a rough time, especially if you've lived a rather sedentary lifestyle up until now. Even the HIIT workouts that claim to be for beginners are going to be difficult for someone who's spent a good portion of their adult life sitting behind a desk or on the couch.

That's not to say it can't be done. Where there's a will, there's a way and some people are able to push through until they get used to the harder routines.

Others will make it halfway through their first workout and call it quits, planning on trying again soon, only to wake up so sore the next morning they give up on HIIT for good. You haven't felt pain until you've pushed through a new workout that really digs into muscles you've barely moved for years. A few aches and pains that evening can turn into sharp, stabbing pains in the morning that make each and every step an agonizing ordeal.

The idea behind HIIT is to get in shape, not to needlessly torture yourself. It's best to start off slow and work your way up to the more difficult HIIT sessions. After all, what good is a HIIT session if it puts you out of commission for a week or longer because you're too sore or injured to keep working out?

The rest of the chapter discusses the preparations you should make in order to get ready to start high-intensity training. Making sure you're ready will go a long way

toward ensuring you make it past the first few sessions of
HIIT.

Get a Physical Exam

Before you start HIIT training, it's imperative you make sure you're physically healthy enough for such a vigorous exercise program. Vigorous exercise puts a strain on your entire body, so it's important to ensure your body will be able to handle it in advance of starting a program. The best way to do this is to visit a doctor and let him know your plans. Ask him specifically to examine you to make sure you're physically healthy enough to do HIIT.

It's a good idea to bring a notebook and a pencil to your examination. Write down the questions you plan on asking in advance of the appointment and take notes on pertinent information. It may seem like it'll be easy to remember during the examination, but you don't want to end up racking your brain for answers later on down the road if you don't take notes.

Here are some questions you should ask your doctor at the examination:

Am I physically able to perform high-intensity interval training?

This is the most important question you're going to ask, so pay close attention. Make sure your doctor knows it isn't just interval training; it's *high-intensity* interval training. Your doctor should be able to tell you about any health issues you have that will preclude you from this sort of training and should be able to provide guidance as to any limitations you may have. Previous or current injuries, illnesses, diseases and/or accidents may make HIIT too difficult or dangerous to perform.

Do I have any medical conditions that limit my ability to do vigorous exercise? Will I make these conditions worse by performing HIIT?

You're looking to get in shape and making current medical conditions worse is not going to help you achieve that goal. If HIIT isn't for you, your doctor should be able to help you choose a more appropriate plan or be willing to refer you to someone who can.

Are there any restrictions as to the actions I can perform? Am I taking any medications that could affect my heart rate?

Take heed of your doctor's advice when it comes to restrictions. Your doctor should be able to provide you with a list of your limitations in light of your current physical condition. Ask your doctor to provide you with a target heart rate you should reach during your workouts and for a danger zone heart rate at which you should stop working out or slow down until your heart drops to a safer level. Be aware that medications that affect your heart rate may make it difficult to use heart rate as an effective metric for measuring vigorous exercise.

Do I need to lose weight? If so, how much?

Here's another important question. Some people overestimate the amount of weight they need to lose, while others underestimate it. Your doctor should be able to give you a good idea of what a reasonable weight loss goal would be and how fast you should be trying to reach that goal.

How is my current weight affecting my health?

This question is more for motivation than anything else. If you doctor tells you you're overweight and your current weight is dangerous to your health, you should be concerned enough about your health to make the changes he or she recommends. While you're at it, ask how much weight you need to lose to improve your health. You might be surprised at how much of a difference a few pounds can make.

Learn How to Monitor Exercise Intensity

In order for HIIT to work its wonders, you have to be able to push yourself hard for short periods of time. How hard you push during these short bursts of exercise can make a big difference in the overall effectiveness of your workouts. **Exercise intensity** is a measurement of how hard you're working and it directly correlates to calories burned, strength gains and changes in weight, body fat and endurance.

There are a number of ways to monitor exercise intensity and some are more effective than others. When you're first starting off, even light exercise may feel intense. You aren't used to the way working out makes you feel and your body hasn't had time to adjust to your new healthy lifestyle, so you're going to feel tired rather quickly. This will change as you gain experience and your body adjusts to the exercises you're doing. Within just a few days your body will start to change.

As you gain experience and get used to HIIT, you'll need to adjust the intensity of your workouts to keep up with the gains in strength and endurance you're realizing. Don't get stuck on a certain length of time, number of exercises or amount of weight. Your HIIT routine should constantly evolve to match your current physical condition. A routine that feels mind-numbingly difficult today will be way too easy a month or two down the road.

You're going to have to constantly adjust your workouts based on your ability to push your body to its limits. In order to do that, you're going to need to know how to tell when you're nearing your limits. The rest of this section lays out methods you can use to measure exertion.

Perceived Exertion

Perceived exertion is the technical term for how tired you feel after a certain set of actions. It's measured on a sliding scale from 1 to 10, with 1 being little to no exertion being felt after completing an exercise and 10 being complete and utter exhaustion.

When it comes to HIIT, you want to push yourself to a high level of perceived exertion during the intense training sessions and then back off to a manageable level during the active recovery sessions. During the high-intensity intervals you should be reaching somewhere in the range of 8 to 10 on the perceived exertion scale. Beginners should shoot for the 5 to 7 range to start. As you improve and become an intermediate exerciser, the 8 to 9 range may be more appropriate. Elite athletes can push themselves closer to 10.

Here's a chart that shows the different levels of perceived exertion:

Exertion	Difficulty
10	Exhaustion
9	Near Exhaustion
8	Very Difficult
7	Difficult
6	Somewhat Difficult
5	Average
4	Fairly Easy

3	Easy
2	Very Easy
1	At Rest

Perceived exertion is highly subjective because some people feel fully exerted long before others will. This isn't necessarily a bad thing, because it's an individualized measurement of how tired you feel. Perceived exertion can vary from day to day and even from hour to hour dependent upon a number of external factors. It is the easiest way to measure how hard you're pushing yourself, since all it requires is being conscious of what your body is telling you—and trust when I say you'll be explicitly aware of how tired you are during a HIIT session.

You should be pushing yourself hard, but not quite to the point where you feel dizzy and are about to pass out. If you're reaching that point, you're probably taking it too far.

The **Talk Test** is sometimes used by those seeking to measure perceived exertion. This is a measurement of how easy it is to talk after engaging in a series of exercises. The ability to speak easily indicates low exertion, while difficulty speaking because of shortness of breath indicates higher exertion.

Target Heart Rate

Stick around the world of HIIT long enough and you'll come across literature that states you don't need to wear a heart rate monitor when you start HIIT because heart rate can't accurately be measured during a HIIT session. The reason for this is there is a lag between your heart rate and the stress your body is being placed under. It's difficult to judge exertion during short intervals by heart rate because your heart rate may not max out until you're in one of your rest periods.

This could end up being very dangerous advice.

The main reason to monitor heart rate isn't to judge when to start and stop exercises. It's to make sure your heart rate doesn't spike up to dangerous levels during the intense exercise periods associated with HIIT. Yes, heart rate does lag a bit behind, but if you hit an extremely high heart rate during exercise, you'll know it's time to back off and enter a rest period earlier than planned, since you know your heart rate might keep climbing after you enter the active recovery period.

It's understandable why some people aren't worried about heart rate during HIIT. For most healthy people, heart rate isn't going to be an issue. Your body will wear down before your heart climbs into dangerous territory and stays there.

Monitoring heart rate during HIIT is largely a precautionary tactic and it's difficult to use it as a measurement of when to start and stop intervals, but there is one good use for heart rate.

It can be useful in judging how hard you're pushing yourself. Your heart rate is a good way to measure how close you're pushing your body to its aerobic and anaerobic thresholds.

In order to use heart rate as a metric, you're going to need to know your **resting heart rate (RHR)**, which is the number of times your heart beats per minute while your body is at rest. Generally speaking, lower numbers indicate better cardiovascular fitness. The normal range for healthy adults is between 60 and 100 beats per minute. Elite athletes can have heart rates that are closer to 40 beats per minute and some may even drop below 30, but it's extremely rare. If you aren't an elite athlete and your heart rate is consistently below 60, it's time to get in to see a doctor. You should also consult with your doctor if your heart rate is consistently above 100.

The best time to check your resting heart rate is in the morning, as soon as you wake up. Your body has been at rest all night and this is the time you're most likely to get an accurate reading. Once you've gotten out of bed and have started moving around, your heart rate will go up.

Here are three easy ways you can check your resting heart rate when you wake up in the morning:

- Place your middle and index fingers onto your wrist, just below your thumb on the inside of your wrist and count the number of beats in a minute.
- Place your middle and index fingers under your jawbone, at the base of where your neck and jaw

meet. Slide your fingers below your jaw to the hollowed out area beside your Adam's apple. Press gently and you should feel your pulse.

- Attach a heart rate monitor and record the number of beats per minute.

Of the three methods, the heart rate monitor is the most accurate, but you can get a pretty good idea of your resting heart rate using the other two.

When using your fingers to check your pulse, either count the number of beats in a full minute or count the number of times your heart beats in 15 seconds and multiply it by 4. Don't use fingers other than your middle and index finger because they can have a pulse of their own, which will throw off your count...and may scare the heck out of you. The first time I took my pulse, I recorded a whopping 120 beats per minute. I used the wrong finger and was counting double. When I checked my pulse the right way, it went down to 70 beats per minute.

For a more accurate picture of your resting heart rate, take a measurement every morning for a week. Add all of the measurements together and divide them by 7 and you'll have a clearer picture of what your average resting heart rate is.

Keep in mind there are a number of factors that can affect resting heart rate. Here are some of the factors that must be taken into consideration:

- **Activity level.**
- **Body position (standing, lying, sitting, etc.).**
- **Health issues.**

- **Illness.**
- **Medications.**
- **Stress and other emotions.**
- **Temperature.**

Once you have your resting heart rate, it's time to figure out your **heart rate reserve (HRR)**. This is the range of heart rates your body is capable of achieving. We already know your resting heart rate, so we'll set that as the low end of the reserve.

Here's an easy method you can use to estimate your **maximum heart rate (MHR)**, which is a measurement of the highest heart rate your body is capable of. All you have to do is subtract your age from 220. Here's the formula:

MHR = 220 – (Your Age)

If your age is 36, you'd subtract 36 from 220 and end up with a maximum heart rate of 184.

While this method is quick and easy, it doesn't take non-age related factors into account. A 36-year old who is in tip-top shape could have a vastly different maximum heart rate than a 36-year old who is overweight and out of shape. To get a more accurate estimate of maximum heart rate, you can pay to take a **graded exercise test**, which is a test of your physical abilities. You'll be asked to perform some sort of fitness test while hooked up to any number of machines. At the end of the test, a printout will be provided that will reveal a number of metrics regarding your level of fitness. If your doctor doesn't offer graded exercise tests, ask to be referred to a clinic or medical center has them on offer.

To figure out your heart rate reserve with the information you now have on hand, subtract your resting heart rate from your maximum heart rate, as follows:

HRR = (Maximum Heart Rate) – (Resting Heart Rate)

Say the 36-year old in the previous example has a resting heart rate of 72 beats per minute and we already figured out he has a maximum heart rate of 184. We plug this information into the heart rate reserve formula, as follows:

HRR = 184 – 72

HRR = 112

This person's estimated heart rate reserve is 112. This number is useful because we can use the **Karvonen formula** to determine the intensity percentage of your heart rate reserve at which you should be working out.

Here is the Karvonen formula:

Training heart rate = (HRR x Intensity Percentage) + RHR

The lower boundary of the intensity percentage will be 50%. Let's plug the information we already have from the previous example into the formula:

Training HR = (HRR x 50%) + RHR

Training HR = (112 x .5) + 72

Training HR = (112 x .5) + 72

Training HR = 128

This is the lower boundary of your target heart rate percentage. 128 beats per minute is the estimated heart rate that will be reached when this person is working at 50% capacity. Training at this heart rate won't do much good.

Next, we need to figure out the training heart rate at 60%, 70%, 80% and 90% using the same formula we just used. Here's a chart showing the training heart rates at each intensity percentage for the 36-year old we've been using as an example:

Intensity Percentage	Heart Rate
50%	128
60%	139
70%	150
80%	167
90%	173

If you don't feel like doing all of the calculations yourself, you can determine your resting heart rate and plug it into an online calculator that does all the work for you. Here are a couple sites you can use:

http://www.briancalkins.com/HeartRate.htm

http://www.sparkpeople.com/resource/calculator_target.asp

Once you have your percentages figured out, you'll have a rough idea of the heart rate zones you want to get into. Beginners will probably want to push themselves into the 50% to 70% range during intervals when first starting off.

Intermediate exercisers may decide to shoot for 70% to 85% during intervals and elite athletes can push themselves to 90%. Start off slow and work your way up to the more intense intervals as you feel your body can handle them. As you gain experience, you can push yourself harder and harder until you're able to get into the higher zones.

It helps to remember that working too hard in the beginning can lead to injury and you'll burn out quickly. On the flip side of the coin, not working hard enough will result in less than stellar gains.

Keep in mind that target heart rates are estimates. Beginners may feel comfortable working at a higher intensity. If you finish a workout feeling like you didn't get anything accomplished, you may need to up the intensity the next time you do a HIIT routine. On the other hand, if you're so tired you can barely move and are still exhausted a day later, you may want to tone things down a bit. It's all about finding a happy medium and constantly adjusting your workouts in order to stay in the zone.

Check with your doctor as to the intensity percentage he or she thinks you should be reaching during HIIT. Take heed of any exercise restrictions your doctor places on you. Certain medications and medical conditions can affect your heart rate and may make it impossible to use your heart rate as a measurement of exercise intensity.

As an example, consider someone taking **beta-blockers**, which are a class of drugs used to reduce stress on the heart in order to treat hypertension, angina, abnormal heart rhythms or any of a number of other medical conditions. High-intensity exercise won't have the same effect on the rhythm of the heart when beta-blockers are in use, so this isn't a good measurement of exercise intensity. A person taking beta-blockers will have to use perceived exertion and/or the Talk Test in order to determine how intensely they're working out.

If you're out of shape and you find your heart rate spiking higher than it should be during or just after intervals, consult with your doctor immediately, as there may be underlying health conditions you aren't aware of that could be putting you in danger when you work out.

Set Goals

If you've made a commitment to losing weight and/or getting fit through HIIT, the best way to ensure you stay on track is to set measurable goals. Without goals, it's easy to start skipping workouts and cheating on your diet. After all, it's tough to stay focused when you aren't holding yourself accountable for your actions.

You've already got the hardest part out of the way. Most people spend more time choosing their workout plan than they do setting their weight loss goals and working toward achieving them. The fact that you've purchased this book is a big step in the right direction. Now it's time to set some realistic and measurable goals that will help further your agenda.

While researching weight loss programs and goals, you may come across a set of standard guidelines for losing weight. These may or may not be a good fit for you, based upon your current health, diet and personal ability. Your doctor and/or a personal trainer should be able to help guide you in the right direction when it comes to setting attainable goals. Don't for a second feel like you have to be shoehorned into set standards. You're an individual and your body may be wired differently than the average person the standard is designed for.

A general guideline for healthy weight loss is one to two pounds per week. Slow weight loss is believed to be better than rapid weight loss because you're more likely to be able to sustain slow weight loss over a long period of time. Rapid weight loss is usually water loss and isn't sustainable. Once the water is gone, the body will go into conservation mode and your metabolism will slow. Weight loss will stop or slow to a crawl and you'll end up frustrated and stuck at a plateau.

We've all heard the saying, "Slow and steady wins the race." This appears to hold true when it comes to weight loss and staying fit as well. What it doesn't hold true for is the high-intensity intervals you'll be doing. Those should be done as fast as you can safely do them.

In order for weight loss goals to work, they have to be measurable. Setting a goal of "I want to lose weight this year" will be significantly less effective than setting a goal that states "I want to lose 40 pounds in 12 months' time." The second goal is a specific goal that allows you to further build upon your weight loss goals by breaking them down into manageable short-term goals. In order to lose 40 pounds in a year, you have to lose just over ¾ of a pound per week. While 40 pounds may sound like a lot, ¾ of a pound per week is manageable for most people.

Setting short-term goals allows you to adjust the intensity of your workouts and your diet if you consistently aren't reaching your short-term goals. A week or two of missed goals aren't a big deal, as long as you're making the adjustments necessary to ensure you don't consistently miss short-term goals. If you only set long-term goals and end up missing them, you could potentially end up wasting *years* of time instead of weeks.

This is one of the biggest pitfalls people find themselves stuck in. The new year rolls around and they declare they're going to start eating healthier, exercising and will lose the extra pounds they've packed on. They work at it for a month or two before getting side-tracked and losing interest because they either aren't seeing the results they expected or they don't feel like working out and eating right anymore. They tell themselves they've got plenty of time to reach their goal before next year gets here. Before they know it, the next year rolls around and the same thing happens. Then the next year . . . and the next year . . . and so on and so forth.

Soon, instead of a few years' worth of extra pounds packed on they've got decades worth of poor diet and lack of exercise to contend with. The body might be able to hold up under the constant bombardment of bad food and bad fitness in the short-term, but it eventually begins to fall apart.

Setting realistic goals will help you avoid the pitfall of "I'll do it this year." You're going to need to set short-term goals that you'll have to make a conscious decision to ignore. Weekly goals allow you to hold yourself accountable every single week. If you're consistently not hitting your weekly goals, you're going to be painfully aware of it.

Of course, you have to set your weight loss goals based on your current weight. If you weigh 220 pounds, then 40 pounds in a year may be reasonable. On the other hand, if you weigh 120 pounds, you're probably going to kill yourself trying to drop 40 pounds. At this point, weight loss probably isn't desirable. It would be time to start setting other fitness goals, like building endurance and improving fitness.

Once the weight loss goals have been set, try to lock in a workout schedule. While you may be tempted to workout 5 to 7 days a week, HIIT training is tough on the body and you should shoot for at least one day off between training sessions. Set an initial goal of three sessions a week and give yourself at least a day off between each session. If you want to work out more than that, you can, but be sure to choose other workout routines that don't involve HIIT.

When setting goals you also have to take any health issues you have into consideration. Diabetics and people with high blood pressure will need to set goals that are different from those who are healthy, especially when it comes to diet. Patients with arthritis and degenerative diseases won't be able to lift as much or push as hard as those who have healthy bones and muscles.

There's a lot to take into consideration, so don't be afraid to get advice from professionals in the field of fitness and health. Your doctor may be able to help, but I'd take it a step further and also talk to a dietician and a personal trainer. They'll be able to give you more targeted advice and are more likely to be able to guide you in the right direction when it comes to setting goals.

Create a Plan

Now that you've got your goals worked out, you've got to design a plan to help you reach those goals. A goal is only as good as the plan that supports it, so this is one of the most important steps you'll take. The more planning you do, the more likely it becomes that you'll achieve your goals.

There are two plans you're going to need to create in order to ensure success:

- **Workout plan.**
- **Diet plan.**

We'll cover workout planning in a bit, but for now it's important to realize you should have your workouts planned well in advance. When you say you're going to work out three times a week whenever you have the time to work out, you're giving yourself an easy exit route whenever you don't feel like working out. It's all too easy to find other "urgent" issues that need to be taken care of instead of working out.

As far as diet planning goes, the best diet plans lay out meals well in advance. Creating a weekly, monthly or even yearly diet plan allows you to plan healthy meals and to purchase the items you'll need in order to make these meals in advance. Don't fall into the trap of saying, "I'm going to start eating healthy this week" without detailing exactly how you're going to eat healthy. You'll find yourself saying the same thing week after week, but taking little action in regard to actually eating healthy.

Plan every last detail, down to the snacks you're going to eat during the day. Planning three meals a day is easy, but good eating habits can seriously be hampered by a trip or two to the vending machine in the middle of day. Plan to eat healthy snacks and you'll be well-ahead of the curve when it comes to weight loss.

Don't use dining out as an excuse to eat unhealthy foods and gorge yourself. The occasional cheat meal as a reward won't do too much damage, but if you eat out all the time, you're going to need to plan your meals while dining out as well. Most restaurants have menus available online, so scope them out in advance and figure out what you're going to eat when dining out.

The crux of your diet plan should be the meals you're eating at home. Breakfast, lunch and dinner should all consist of whole, healthy foods that will make you healthier, as opposed to hampering your fitness efforts. Figure out what you're going to eat for each meal during the week and write it down.

Pick one day during the week as your shopping day and create a list of all the foods you're going to need based on your meal plan. The less time you spend at the grocery store, the better. Once you start eating healthy, you'll be amazed at the row after row of unhealthy food you now have to traverse to get to the good stuff. There's temptation around every corner (and on most of the end displays), so get in, get what you need for the week and get out, hopefully without having tossed anything unhealthy in the cart.

One trick you can use at most grocery stores is to stick to the perimeter of the store. This is where most of the healthy foods will be. You'll still have to ignore some unhealthy foods, but the middle aisles are usually packed full of processed and unhealthy foods.

While a full-scale diet plan is beyond the scope of this book, there is a ton of resources out there, both paid and free diet plans being a Google search away. Create a diet plan and stick to it and you'll be well on your way to reaching your weight loss goals. HIIT will be the icing on the cake that tones your body and kicks your weight loss effort into high gear.

HIIT for Beginners

Most workout programs shoehorn both beginners and veterans into the same workout plan, leaving the beginners sweating profusely, out of breath and cursing the workout instructor as they gasp for air just minutes into the routine. Little regard is given to those who are just getting started, unless you're working with a personal trainer who's willing to ease you in.

When I first started working out, I was about 50 pounds overweight. I'd tricked myself into believing I was in halfway decent shape, even though the only thing I'd been consistently curling for the previous ten years were bottles of beer. I proudly purchased the Insanity workout program and told my family and friends I'd decided it was time to get in shape. I was filled with trepidation the day the package arrived in the mail and I eagerly opened it and popped the DVD into the DVD player. I skipped ahead to the first workout, eager to start my fitness journey.

I made it to the one minute mark before I realized I was in serious trouble. I was gassed by the 5 minute mark, but still somehow managed to barely mimic what I saw onscreen until 10 full minutes had passed. I hadn't even made it out of the warm-ups and sweat was pouring off me in buckets as I gasped for breath. I collapsed onto the couch and watched the rest of the workout, wondering if I'd somehow managed to skip ahead to the advanced level. I looked on in amazement as the people on screen bounced and jumped and stretched their way through the workout with ease.

I woke up the next day sore and tired, but determined to give it another go. Once again, I barely got past the warm-up exercise before I was too exhausted to continue and collapsed on the couch. To this day (and much to my wife's chagrin), there's a sweat ring on the couch where I flopped down the second day. I fell asleep before the routine was finished and slept a good five or six hours straight.

I woke up to excruciating pain. It felt like I'd torn every muscle in my body. My legs were cramped to the point where trying to stretch them and move them sent bolts of pain shooting through my body. My back, chest and torso throbbed with pain and to top things off, I had a pounding headache. I didn't work out again for three months. Not because I was injured, as it only took a week to recover. The rest of the time was spent pondering whether I really wanted to put myself through that level of extreme torture again.

If you're out of shape and are looking to get back into a shape other than round, go easy until you're ready to push yourself to the limit. If the workouts in future chapters are too taxing, and many of them will be since HIIT is designed for athletes, cut the workout in half or even by a third by shortening the duration of the intervals. Once you're able to make it through the shortened routine, slowly but surely increase the time of the intervals until you're up to the 20 minute mark. There's no need to torture yourself and you may end up doing more harm than good if you try to start with the longer, harder HIIT workouts.

As you perform a workout routine, monitor your heart rate and perceived exhaustion and move on to more difficult workouts as you're able to. You're the best judge of what you're capable of and you'll soon find yourself knocking the tougher workouts out of the park.

When choosing a HIIT routine, the best routine is the one you're able to finish right as you reach the point where you're ready to give up. The whole goal of HIIT is to push yourself as hard as you can for short bursts, followed by active recovery periods where you recover just enough to push yourself hard again.

Buying Running Shoes

A good pair of running shoes is an investment that'll pay dividends in the long run. Ill-fitting, worn-out shoes open you up to injury and place undue stress on your body. You're more likely to stick to a workout routine if you have good shoes that fit comfortably. Nothing kills plans to work out faster than waking up to aching feet that are covered in large blisters.

While you may be tempted to dust off that old pair of sneakers you've had sitting in the closet since you graduated high school, this is one of the worst things you could do. Invest a little money in a good pair of running shoes and your feet will thank you for it by not barking too loud after a good workout.

Here are some tips you can use to ensure you get a good pair of running shoes:

- **Spend a little cash.** Running shoes are one of those areas where you generally get what you pay for. You don't need run out and buy a $220 pair of ECCO BIOM A running shoes (unless you really want to) when you're first getting started. If you're willing to spend around $100, you can get a solid pair of running shoes that'll serve you well. Go too cheap on the shoes and your feet will remind you of it every step of the way.

- **Talk to other runners before buying a pair of shoes.** Check with people you know who run to see what shoes they prefer. If you have a specialty running store close to where you live, the advice you get from experts there could be invaluable. When all else fails, hit the running forums on the Internet. Just be ready to see a lot of arguing over which brand makes the better shoe.

- **Get the right fit.** It doesn't matter how good the shoe is if it doesn't fit properly. Even the best shoes will rub your feet raw if they're too loose or will leave you in pain if they're too tight. Don't be afraid to jog around the store, as long as it isn't too crowded. You might get some strange looks, but that's a small price to pay to get shoes that fit your feet properly.

- **Don't order shoes online.** Unless you know exactly what you want and what size to order, you'll be much better off going to the store to purchase your shoes in person. Even if you're sure you know what to buy, it's a lot easier to return shoes to a brick-and-mortar store than it is to some fly-by-night Internet store you hunted down to save a few bucks.

- **Wear the same socks you'll be wearing while exercising.** Wearing different socks can make shoes feel completely different. Be sure to wear the same socks you'll be wearing while running or exercising.

- **Don't wear your shoes out.** Shoes start to break down long before they start to fall apart. Replace your shoes regularly to keep your feet in good shape.

- **Listen to what your body is telling you.** If your feet, legs, shins or knees are hurting or aching more than usual, this may be a sign your midsoles are wearing down. Keep wearing the same shoes and the little problems you're suffering now could turn into much bigger problems that leave you sitting on the sidelines.

You'll get a lot of advice when it comes to picking the right pair of shoes, but you're ultimately the one who's going to have to wear them. If you try on a pair of shoes that's been getting rave reviews and it doesn't feel right to you, look for a pair that does feel right. Everybody's feet are different and what's perfect for one person may be constant misery for another.

Creating a Workout Plan

Think of your workout plan as a roadmap to a stronger and healthier body. The more complete your road map is, the less likely you are to get hopelessly lost along the way.

The first item on the agenda is figuring out what days of the week you're going to work out. In order to realize maximum benefit, HIIT shouldn't be done two days in a row, so the most HIIT workouts you're going to want to do in a week is four. You can start on Sunday, take Monday off, workout Tuesday, take Wednesday off and continue alternating days like this until the end of the week.

Your fourth workout of the week will be on Sunday, so you'll have to take Monday off the next week and will only be able to get three workouts in the second week, alternating a day between each workout. Here's a sample 4-week schedule with the days you'd be working out shaded in gray:

Mo	Tu	We	Th	Fr	Sa	Su
Mo	Tu	We	Th	Fr	Sa	Su
Mo	Tu	We	Th	Fr	Sa	Su
Mo	Tu	We	Th	Fr	Sa	Su

Four HIIT sessions a week are a lot for most people. You might decide you only want to work out three days a week. When you use this schedule, you have a little more flexibility in picking the days you work out. Here's a sample plan showing only 3 days a week:

Mo	Tu	We	Th	Fr	Sa	Su
Mo	Tu	We	Th	Fr	Sa	Su
Mo	Tu	We	Th	Fr	Sa	Su
Mo	Tu	We	Th	Fr	Sa	Su

Beginners might want to only workout twice a week. If you aren't in good shape, your first few HIIT workouts are going to be rough. Scheduling them twice a week for the first month may be required to give your body enough time to recover for the next workout.

Here's a sample plan in which you'd only work out twice a week:

Mo	Tu	We	Th	Fr	Sa	Su
Mo	Tu	We	Th	Fr	Sa	Su
Mo	Tu	We	Th	Fr	Sa	Su
Mo	Tu	We	Th	Fr	Sa	Su

On your days off, you can either take a break to give your sore and tired body time to recover or you can engage in light exercise like a brisk walk through the neighborhood or some light cardio. Bodybuilders may decide they want to lift on days they aren't doing HIIT.

The key to creating a workout plan is building one you're going to be able to stick to. If you know your boss almost always asks you to work late on Thursdays and Fridays, don't schedule workout days on those days unless you're really planning on hitting the gym after a long day at work.

If you have kids, you'll either have to have daycare lined up (unless you're lucky enough to be a member at a gym that offers daycare) or you're going to have to plan workouts that can be done at home. The good thing about HIIT is you don't need a gym. There are plenty of exercises you can do in the comfort of your living room or in your backyard.

Once you've got a schedule worked out, it's time to choose your HIIT workouts. There are a bunch of them you can choose from, many of which are covered in later chapters in the book. You can choose one HIIT workout and try to push yourself a little harder each time or you can select a variety of workouts, maybe doing sprinting one day a week, weight training another day of the week and body weight training the third day you work out.

Choosing a workout plan is a highly individual experience. Some people prefer a variety of workouts and enjoy doing different things all the time, while others like to do a single type of workout and are driven by constantly pushing themselves to new personal records.

It doesn't matter what you pick. What matters is picking something you're going to be able to stick with for the long haul. For most people, this means switching things up every once in a while so they don't fall into a rut. If you find you've reached a plateau and don't seem to be losing any more weight, try switching routines. A simple change like this may be all it takes to shock your body into burning fat again.

Interval Ratios

When you start researching HIIT workouts, you'll probably come across a number of recommendations as to what the proper ratio of work to active recovery is. This ratio is usually presented in the following format:

Work : Rest

The work part of the ratio refers to the high-intensity intervals and the rest part of the ratio refers to the active recovery periods. A ratio of 1 : 1 would mean for every period of work, there would be an equal active recovery period. If your high-intensity interval lasts 1 minute, your active recovery period would be 1 minute as well. If your high-intensity interval lasts 30 seconds, your rest period would also be 30 seconds.

Novice exercisers should start off at a 1 : 3 or even a 1 : 4 work to rest ratio. What this means is for every period of time spent in an intense interval, 3 or 4 times that amount of time would be spent in an active recovery period, respectively. If you spend 30 seconds in an intense interval, a 1 : 3 ratio would mean you need to rest for a minute and a half. A 1 : 4 ratio would equate to a 2 minute active recovery period after the same interval.

As you gain experience, work your way up to a 1 : 1 ratio. Once you reach a 1 : 1 ratio, start increasing the length of time of your intervals. If you're doing 30-second intervals, move up to 45-second interval and then 1-minutes intervals and so on.

Regardless of how fit you are, if you're going all-out during the high-intensity intervals, you should finish each and every workout feeling like you gave it everything you've got. The rest periods should be just long enough for you to catch your breath a little and be ready to go all-out again. Don't be afraid to play around with the ratios of work to active recovery until you find yourself in the right zone.

Sprint Interval Training (SIT)

Sprint Interval Training (SIT) is HIIT broken down to its simplest form. All you need is a good pair of running shoes and somewhere open enough to where you'll be able to jog and sprint. It can be done at a neighborhood park, in a school field or even in your backyard, if it's big enough. These routines can also be run on a treadmill, so you can knock them out at the gym, if that's your thing.

Sprint interval training benefits you in that it improves both your muscle power and your stamina. You won't just be faster and fitter. You'll find sprint training will help you in the gym as well. You'll be able to push harder and burn more calories no matter what workout you're doing when you integrate sprint training into your exercise regimen.

A 2011 Canadian study found that a 6-week training program consisting of 4 to 6 30-second sprints followed by a 4-minute recovery period helped participants lose 12.4% of their body fat. A separate group of participants who were asked to participate in an endurance training program lost less than half that amount. The sprint group spent less than an hour running while the endurance group spent more than 13 hours running (7). This appears to indicate the training time required to lose weight via HIIT is much, much less than it is with endurance training or steady-state cardio.

Basic SIT

With SIT, you'll warm up by walking or jogging at a light pace for 5 minutes. After the warm-up period, increase your jogging speed and jog at a slightly faster pace for 2 minutes. Next, sprint as fast as you can for 30 seconds. Follow that up with a 2-minute jogging session, followed by another 30-second sprint. Continue the jogging/sprinting intervals for 20 minutes and then cool down by walking or jogging at a moderate pace for 3 to 5 minutes.

Here's the breakdown of this basic workout:

Time	Exercise	Exertion (1 - 10)
5 minutes	Warm up. Light walking or jogging.	3 to 5
2 minutes	Moderate walking or jogging.	5 to 6
30 seconds	Full-speed sprint.	8 to 9
2 minutes	Moderate walking or jogging.	5 to 6
30 seconds	Full-speed sprint.	8 to 9
2 minutes	Moderate walking or jogging.	5 to 6
30 seconds	Full-speed sprint.	8 to 9
2 minutes	Moderate walking or jogging.	5 to 6
30 seconds	Full-speed sprint.	8 to 9
Repeat the intervals one more time for a total of 20 minutes of intervals.		

| 5 minutes | Cool down. Moderate walking or jogging. | 3 to 5 |

Beginners may want to cut the sprints in this workout down to 15 seconds. It doesn't sound like much, but 15 seconds of running at full speed will be exhausting if you're out of shape. As your cardiovascular ability and endurance improves, you'll be able to step up the length and intensity of the full-speed sprints while decreasing the active recovery periods.

The intervals in the previous routine use a 1 : 4 intensity ratio. If this is too easy, try changing the interval intensity ration.

Here's a breakdown of a more difficult SIT workout that uses a 1 :3 ratio:

Time	Exercise	Exertion (1 - 10)
5 minutes	Warm up. Light walking or jogging.	3 to 5
1 minute, 30 seconds	Moderate walking or jogging.	5 to 6
30 seconds	Full-speed sprint.	8 to 9
1 minute, 30 seconds	Moderate walking or jogging.	5 to 6
30 seconds	Full-speed sprint.	8 to 9
1 minute, 30 seconds	Moderate walking or jogging.	5 to 6
30 seconds	Full-speed sprint.	8 to 9

1 minute, 30 seconds	Moderate walking or jogging.	5 to 6
30 seconds	Full-speed sprint	8 to 9
1 minute, 30 seconds	Moderate walking or jogging.	5 to 6
30 seconds	Full-speed sprint.	8 to 9
Repeat the intervals one more time for a total of 20 minutes of intervals.		
5 minutes	Cool down. Moderate walking or jogging.	3 to 5

The only thing that changed is the interval times for the active recovery periods were decreased.

To make things even tougher, you could play around with the interval times and shorten the duration of the active recovery periods, as follows:

Time	Exercise	Exertion (1 - 10)
5 minutes	Warm up. Light walking or jogging.	3 to 5
2 minutes	Moderate walking or jogging.	5 to 6
1 minute	Full-speed sprint.	8 to 9
2 minutes	Moderate walking or jogging.	5 to 6
1 minute	Full-speed sprint.	8 to 9

2 minutes	Moderate walking or jogging.	5 to 6
1 minute	Full-speed sprint.	8 to 9
Repeat intervals a second time. The interval portion of this workout will take approximately 18 minutes.		
5 minutes	Cool down. Moderate walking or jogging.	3 to 5

This workout has a 1 : 2 work to rest ratio and will be difficult for all but the most experienced of exercisers and athletes.

Pyramid SIT

If you're looking for an even tougher workout, try a pyramid sprint session. **Pyramid sessions** ramp up the difficulty by increasing the sprint time from interval to interval until the middle of the workout, at which time they reverse the time spent sprinting until the sprint intervals drop back down to the interval time you started at.

Here's a pyramid sprint interval workout that'll really test your endurance:

Time	Exercise	Exertion (1 - 10)
5 minutes	Warm up. Light walking or jogging.	3 to 5
30 seconds	Full-speed sprint.	8 to 9
1 minute	Moderate walking or jogging.	5 to 6
1 minute	Full-speed sprint.	8 to 9
2 minutes	Moderate walking or jogging.	5 to 6
2 minutes	Full-speed sprint.	8 to 9
4 minutes	Moderate walking or jogging.	5 to 6
1 minute	Full-speed sprint.	8 to 9
2 minutes	Moderate walking or jogging.	5 to 6
30 seconds	Full-speed sprint.	8 to 9
1 minute	Moderate walking or jogging.	5 to 6
5 minutes	Cool down. Moderate walking or jogging.	3 to 5

This pyramid is brutal and is best left to the elite athletes. 2-minute sprints start to push the limits of the cardiovascular system, so keep a close eye on your heart rate and back off or shorten the duration of the sprint if it gets too high.

Variable Distance SIT

Yet another way to do sprint intervals is to vary the distance you're running for each of the sprints. Start with a 100-meter sprint and work your way up to 400 meters, increasing the distance by 100 meters every time you sprint.

This is what the workout would look like:

Time	Exercise	Exertion (1 - 10)
5 minutes	Warm up. Light walking or jogging.	3 to 5
Not applicable	100-meter sprint.	8 to 9
3 minutes	Light walking or jogging.	3 to 5
Not applicable	200-meter sprint.	8 to 9
3 minutes	Light walking or jogging.	3 to 5
Not applicable	300-meter sprint.	8 to 9
3 minutes	Light walking or jogging.	3 to 5
Not applicable	400-meter sprint.	8 to 9
3 minutes	Light walking or jogging.	3 to 5
5 minutes	Cool down. Light walking or jogging.	3 to 5

A 2011 study of healthy elite handball players between the ages of 17 and 25 had a group of them participate in a similar conditioning routine run on a treadmill. The sprints were run at 80% of their maximum speed. The interval training sessions led to elevated lactate, growth hormone and testosterone levels, which are all indicative of an effective workout routine (8).

SIT for Wrestlers and MMA Fighters

Wrestlers need to be in peak condition come competition time and this condition must be sustained throughout the season. Cardiovascular condition and strength are both integral components of a wrestler's game.

A recent study showed sprint interval training to be an effective means of preparing for wrestling season because it improved anaerobic conditioning and strength at the same time. Each wrestler who participated in the experimental group in the study ran sets of six 35-meter sprints with a 10-second recovery time between each sprint. The SIT routine was performed twice a week for 4 weeks as part of an overall conditioning and training routine. The experimental group showed significant improvements in cardiovascular ability, peak power output and mean power output after the study. Total testosterone increased significantly as well (9).

Here's a workout you can use to get similar results. This SIT workout may be a good option for wrestlers, MMA fighters and others who are seeking to maximize gains in both strength and endurance by adding a HIIT workout to their normal conditioning routines.

Time	Exercise	Exertion (1 - 10)
5 minutes	Warm up. Light walking or jogging.	3 to 5
Not applicable	35-meter sprint.	8 to 9
10 seconds	Active recovery.	1 to 3

Not applicable	35-meter sprint.	8 to 9
10 seconds	Active recovery.	1 to 3
Not applicable	35-meter sprint.	8 to 9
10 seconds	Active recovery.	1 to 3
Not applicable	35-meter sprint.	8 to 9
10 seconds	Active recovery.	1 to 3
Not applicable	35-meter sprint.	8 to 9
10 seconds	Active recovery.	1 to 3
Not applicable	35-meter sprint.	8 to 9
10 seconds	Active recovery.	1 to 3
5 minutes	Cool down. Light walking or jogging.	3 to 5

If one set of six sprints isn't enough, repeat the six sets of 35-meter sprints as many times as you feel comfortable. Keep a close eye on your heart rate and watch your perceived exertion. You've got to be careful not to overdo it with this routine.

SIT for Athletes

If you're an athlete training for a sport that requires quick bursts of explosive movement followed by lulls in the action (think basketball or baseball), you may be better served by an unpredictable workout that mixes things up. You can mix and match the distance or time of your sprints and you can shorten and lengthen your rest periods. This can be done however you'd like.

Here's an example of how a mix-and-match session might look:

Time	Exercise	Exertion (1 - 10)
5 minutes	Warm up. Light walking or jogging.	3 to 5
30 seconds	Full-speed sprint.	8 to 9
2 minutes	Moderate walking or jogging.	5 to 6
1 minute	Full-speed sprint.	8 to 9
1 minute	Moderate walking or jogging.	5 to 6
45 seconds	Full-speed sprint.	8 to 9
3 minutes	Moderate walking or jogging.	5 to 6
30 seconds	Full-speed sprint.	8 to 9
2 minutes	Moderate walking or jogging.	5 to 6
1 minute	Full-speed sprint.	8 to 9

1 minute	Moderate walking or jogging.	5 to 6
1 minute, 30 seconds	Full-speed sprint.	8 to 9
2 minutes	Moderate walking or jogging.	5 to 6
5 minutes	Cool down. Light walking or jogging.	3 to 5

Don't try to figure out a pattern in the previous workout. There isn't one. Random sprint times have been mixed and matched with active recovery periods to create a workout that keeps the body guessing.

Endurance athletes can up the intensity level of their workouts by running the sprints uphill. Mark off the distance you plan on running and sprint uphill at full speed. Walk or jog your way back down to starting point and sprint again. Repeat this process as soon as you're able to run uphill at 100% again.

Add Other Exercises to Build Muscle

SIT workouts can be combined with body weight workouts like sit-ups and push-ups to build even more strength. Do the sit-ups and/or the push-ups immediately after you finish each sprint.

Here's what a SIT workout would look like when sit-ups and push-ups have been added:

Time	Exercise	Exertion (1 - 10)
5 minutes	Warm up. Light walking or jogging.	3 to 5
Not applicable	100-meter sprint.	8 to 9
Not applicable	15 push-ups.	6 to 8
Not applicable	20 sit-ups.	6 to 8
2 minutes	Light walking or jogging.	3 to 5
Not applicable	100-meter sprint.	8 to 9
Not applicable	15 push-ups.	6 to 8
Not applicable	20 sit-ups.	6 to 8
2 minutes	Light walking or jogging.	3 to 5
Not applicable	100-meter sprint.	8 to 9
Not applicable	15 push-ups.	6 to 8
Not applicable	20 sit-ups.	6 to 8
Repeat intervals until 20 minutes have passed.		

5 minutes	Cool down. Light walking or jogging.	3 to 5

Alternatively, you can add SIT routines to an overall weight training program designed to build muscle. One or two SIT sessions a week will improve your gains in the gym, helping you build strength while keeping those extra inches off your waistline.

A Quick & Easy SIT Workout

Here's a quick and easy HIIT workout I use when I don't feel like keeping track of time. I head out to my local high school and use the boundaries of the football field as a track. I jog around the perimeter of the field once to warm up. I'll then alternate between sprinting the length of the field and jogging the width of the field until I'm too tired to continue.

Alternatively, if you're somewhere that has a track, you can alternate between jogging and sprinting on the track. The easiest way to do this is to jog the curved sections of the track, while sprinting the straight sections. Repeat this as many times as you can.

Exercise Machine HIIT

The HIIT workouts in this section are all done on exercise machines. They can be performed at the gym or by anyone who has an exercise machine at home. The following machines are used in various routines in this chapter:

- **Elliptical.**
- **Stair Stepper.**
- **Stationary Bike.**
- **Treadmill.**

One question people constantly ask me is what resistance (or incline) they should set their machines to. There is no set resistance that everyone should do for HIIT workouts. You should set the resistance or incline on your machine as high as you can set it and still finish the high-intensity intervals at full speed.

Treadmill HIIT

The treadmill is probably the most ubiquitous workout machine in existence. Most gyms have a variety of them and a number of people have them at home. The problem with treadmills is most people use them the same way, and the way they're using them isn't the most effective way to lose weight and stay in shape. Most treadmill users hop on the treadmill and warm up for a while, before setting the treadmill to a constant speed and incline and running or walking for anywhere from 20 minutes to an hour.

HIIT on the treadmill are much more effective than steady-state workouts. A HIIT treadmill workout shocks the body and forces it to start burning body fat for energy.

Most of the sprinting routines from the SIT chapter can easily be converted to treadmill routines. Instead of sprinting as fast as you can across an open area, you'll be sprinting in place on the treadmill. Your intervals will consist of high-intensity sprints coupled with low- to moderate-intensity jogging. The intensity of your running on the treadmill can be adjusted by changing the speed and/or the incline at which you're running.

In addition to speed, the treadmill offers you the added benefit of setting the incline, which simulates walking or running uphill. A 2% incline on the treadmill is supposed to feel similar to walking up a hill with a 2% grade.

In order to get the most benefit from your treadmill routine, you're going to need to have good form. If you're one of those treadmill runners—and many runners are— who keeps a constant grip on the treadmill handrails, it's time to kick that bad habit. Using the treadmill without holding onto it forces your body to use more muscles and helps you keep proper posture during your workout. If you're worried about falling, set the treadmill to a lower speed before releasing your grip for the first time. You'll find it quickly feels natural and you'll be back to your old speed and incline in no time at all.

I've purposely avoided providing set speeds or inclines in these HIIT routines. Set the inclines and the speeds at a level you're comfortable with that'll push your heart rate into the right zone. The right speed and incline will vary from individual to individual. Those who are out of shape will find themselves pushed to the limit by a setting of 1% grade at 1 to 2 miles per hour. Intermediate exercisers can bump the incline up to 3% to 5% and increase speed to 2 to 3 MPH. Elite athletes may be able to workout at a 10% grade or above and speeds in excess of 10 MPH.

Be careful not to set the bar too high or you risk injury. Start slower than you think you'll be able to handle and work your way up to the faster speeds and steeper inclines. Use your heart rate and/or perceived exertion to judge when you're in the right zone. Ideally, HIIT intervals will require everything you've got and you'll be able to recover just enough during the active recovery periods to do it all again during the next high-intensity period.

Here's a basic treadmill routine that keeps the incline the same, but varies the speed during the workout. Set the incline based on your fitness level. Higher inclines will equate to a more difficult workout. As far as speed goes, set the speed high enough to where it's really going to get your heart pumping for the high-intensity portions of the routine and lower it to a light jog or a fast walk for the active recovery periods. Elite athletes may be able to set the incline to 15% or higher and still complete the workout:

Time	Exercise	Exertion (1 - 10)
5 minutes	Warm up. Low speed.	3 to 5
30 seconds	High speed.	8 to 9
1 minute	Low to moderate speed.	5 to 7
Continue alternating between high and low speed until 20 minutes have passed.		
5 minutes	Cool down. Light walking or jogging.	3 to 5

Once you're able to handle this workout with ease, try upping the length of the high-intensity intervals

This workout can be made much more difficult by varying the incline throughout the workout, as follows:

Time	Exercise	Exertion (1 - 10)
5 minutes	Warm up. Low speed.	3 to 5
30 seconds	High speed. Steep incline.	8 to 9
1 minute	Low to moderate speed. Low incline.	5 to 7

Continue alternating between high and low speed and steep and low incline until 20 minutes have passed.		
5 minutes	Cool down. Light walking or jogging.	3 to 5

Here's another routine that varies the incline and the length of the interval times to create a workout that will really put you to the test:

Time	Exercise	Exertion (1 - 10)
5 minutes	Warm up. Low speed.	3 to 5
30 seconds	High speed. Steep incline.	8 to 9
1 minute	Low to moderate speed. Low incline.	5 to 7
1 minute	High speed. Steep incline.	8 to 9
2 minutes	Low to moderate speed. Low incline.	5 to 7
30 seconds	High speed. Steep incline.	8 to 9
1 minute	Low to moderate speed. Low incline.	5 to 7
1 minute	High speed. Steep incline.	8 to 9
2 minutes	Low to moderate speed. Low incline.	5 to 7
30 seconds	High speed. Steep incline.	8 to 9
1 minute	Low to moderate speed.	5 to 7

	Low incline.	
\multicolumn{3}{}{Repeat intervals a second time.}
5 minutes	Cool down. Light walking or jogging.	3 to 5

If you prefer pyramid routines, they can be done on the treadmill as well. Here's a sample pyramid routine to get you started:

Time	Exercise	Exertion (1 - 10)
5 minutes	Warm up. Low speed.	3 to 5
30 seconds	High speed. Steep incline.	8 to 9
30 seconds	Low to moderate speed. Low incline.	5 to 7
45 seconds	High speed. Steep incline.	8 to 9
45 seconds	Low to moderate speed. Low incline.	5 to 7
1 minute	High speed. Steep incline.	8 to 9
1 minute	Low to moderate speed. Low incline.	5 to 7
2 minutes	High speed. Steep incline.	8 to 9
2 minutes	Low to moderate speed. Low incline.	5 to 7
2 minutes	High speed. Steep incline.	8 to 9

2 minutes	Low to moderate speed. Low incline.	5 to 7
1 minute	High speed. Steep incline.	8 to 9
1 minutes	Low to moderate speed. Low incline.	5 to 7
45 seconds	High speed. Steep incline.	8 to 9
45 seconds	Low to moderate speed. Low incline.	5 to 7
30 seconds	High speed. Steep incline.	8 to 9
30 seconds	Low to moderate speed. Low incline.	5 to 7
5 minutes	Cool down. Light walking or jogging.	3 to 5

You'd better be in good shape if you plan on doing this workout. It's a tough one!

Stationary Bicycle HIIT

A 2008 study by the University of South Wales in Australia found that young women who participated in a HIIT program for 15 weeks were able to realize significant reductions in body mass and fasting plasma insulin levels in comparison to a group who engaged in steady-state exercise only.

The women in the high-intensity exercise group exercised three times a week. They alternated between 8 seconds of hard cycling with heavy resistance, followed by 12 seconds of slow pedaling at a light resistance for a maximum of 60 repeats in each session. They started off with session as short as 5 minutes and gradually worked their way up to 20 minutes sessions (10).

To do a similar workout at home, try the following:

Time	Exercise	Exertion (1 - 10)
5 minutes	Warm up. Light cycling.	3 to 5
8 seconds	Cycling full-speed with heavy resistance.	8 to 9
12 seconds	Cycling slowly with light resistance.	5 to 7
Repeat 8-second heavy and 12-second light cycling until 20 minutes have passed.		
5 minutes	Cool down. Light cycling.	3 to 5

While this workout will be tiring for novice exercisers, it may not be enough for experienced exercisers or well-conditioned athletes. If you want to step it up a notch, try changing the heavy resistance intervals to 30-seconds, 45-seconds or even a minute. You'll also want to increase the recovery times to allow your heart rate time to recover a bit before you jump back into the heavy pedaling.

This routine will really up the level of difficulty of this workout.

Time	Exercise	Exertion (1 - 10)
5 minutes	Warm up. Light cycling.	3 to 5
45 seconds	Cycling full-speed with heavy resistance.	8 to 9
1 minute	Cycling slowly with light resistance.	5 to 7
Repeat 45-second heavy and 1-minute light cycling until 20 minutes have passed.		
5 minutes	Cool down. Light cycling.	3 to 5

Pyramid routines also work well when using an exercise bike:

Time	Exercise	Exertion (1 - 10)
5 minutes	Warm up. Light cycling.	3 to 5

15 seconds	Cycling full-speed with heavy resistance.	8 to 9
15 seconds	Cycling slowly with light resistance.	5 to 7
30 seconds	Cycling full-speed with heavy resistance.	8 to 9
30 seconds	Cycling slowly with light resistance.	5 to 7
45 seconds	Cycling full-speed with heavy resistance.	8 to 9
45 seconds	Cycling slowly with light resistance.	5 to 7
1 minute	Cycling full-speed with heavy resistance.	8 to 9
1 minute	Cycling slowly with light resistance.	5 to 7
45 seconds	Cycling full-speed with heavy resistance.	8 to 9
45 seconds	Cycling slowly with light resistance.	5 to 7
30 seconds	Cycling full-speed with heavy resistance.	8 to 9
30 seconds	Cycling slowly with light resistance.	5 to 7
15 seconds	Cycling full-speed with heavy resistance.	8 to 9
15 seconds	Cycling slowly with light resistance.	5 to 7
5 minutes	Cool down. Light cycling.	3 to 5

If this pyramid workout is too easy, cycle through the resistance pyramid more than once or up the time spent during the high-intensity intervals, as follows:

Time	Exercise	Exertion (1 - 10)
5 minutes	Warm up. Light cycling.	3 to 5
1 minute	Cycling full-speed with heavy resistance.	8 to 9
1 minute	Cycling slowly with light resistance.	5 to 7
1 minute	Cycling full-speed with heavy resistance.	8 to 9
1 minute	Cycling slowly with light resistance.	5 to 7
1 minute	Cycling full-speed with heavy resistance.	8 to 9
1 minute	Cycling slowly with light resistance.	5 to 7
2 minutes	Cycling full-speed with heavy resistance.	8 to 9
2 minutes	Cycling slowly with light resistance.	5 to 7
2 minutes	Cycling full-speed with heavy resistance.	8 to 9
2 minutes	Cycling slowly with light resistance.	5 to 7
1 minute	Cycling full-speed with heavy resistance.	8 to 9

1 minute	Cycling slowly with light resistance.	5 to 7
1 minute	Cycling full-speed with heavy resistance.	8 to 9
1 minute	Cycling slowly with light resistance.	5 to 7
1 minute	Cycling full-speed with heavy resistance.	8 to 9
1 minute	Cycling slowly with light resistance.	5 to 7
5 minutes	Cool down. Light cycling.	3 to 5

This workout will give you a full 20-minute HIIT session that should push you to your limits. You may have to reduce the resistance in the high-intensity intervals of the routine in able to allow yourself to push as hard as you can for the entire duration of the interval.

The key to a successful HIIT exercise bike workout is pushing yourself as hard as you can during the heavy resistance phases of the routine. Otherwise, all you're doing is interval training, which is effective in its own right, but isn't exactly HIIT.

Elliptical HIIT

The elliptical trainer is a good choice for those looking for a HIIT workout that's about as low-impact as a HIIT workout can get. Since you never lift your feet off of the trainer, there's no impact and no damage done to your feet every time they hit the ground.

It's important you use the right amount of resistance when using an elliptical trainer. If you're able to get the machine moving fast enough to where you can hear it spinning, you've got the resistance set too low. Instead, bump the resistance up until you have to work at getting the elliptical moving.

When using the elliptical for the following HIIT routine, set the resistance as high as you can handle and leave it there. Push at a moderate pace during the active recovery periods and push as fast as you can during the high-intensity intervals.

Here's a sample elliptical HIIT workout:

Time	Exercise	Exertion (1 - 10)
5 minutes	Warm up. Light resistance. Light pushing.	3 to 5
30 seconds	Heavy resistance. Hard pushing.	8 to 9
1 minute, 30 seconds	Heavy resistance. Moderate pushing.	5 to 7
Repeat 30-second heavy and 30-light pushing until 20		

	minutes have passed.	
5 minutes	Cool down. Low resistance. Light pushing.	3 to 5

This next workout plays around with the resistance during the high-intensity and the active recovery periods:

Time	Exercise	Exertion (1 - 10)
5 minutes	Warm up. Light resistance. Light pushing forward.	3 to 5
1 minute	Heavy resistance. Hard pushing forward.	8 to 9
2 minutes	Light resistance. Moderate pushing forward.	5 to 7
1 minute	Heavy resistance. Hard pushing forward.	8 to 9
2 minutes	Light resistance. Moderate pushing forward.	5 to 7
Repeat intervals until 20 minutes have passed.		
5 minutes	Cool down. Low resistance. Light pushing forward.	3 to 5

Elliptical machines can be run both forward and in reverse. This workout switches back and forth between forward and backward movement on the elliptical:

Time	Exercise	Exertion (1 - 10)
5 minutes	Warm up. Light resistance. Light pushing forward.	3 to 5
1 minute	Heavy resistance. Hard pushing forward.	8 to 9
2 minutes	Heavy resistance. Light pushing forward.	5 to 7
1 minute	Heavy resistance. Hard pushing backward.	8 to 9
2 minutes	Heavy resistance. Light pushing backward.	5 to 7
Repeat intervals until 20 minutes have passed.		
5 minutes	Cool down. Low resistance. Light pushing forward.	3 to 5

Just because the elliptical is low-impact doesn't mean it has to be low-intensity. Find the right combination of resistance and pushing and push yourself to the limit. The heavy resistance sprints should leave you gassed at the end of each one. If not, push harder.

Stair Stepper HIIT

Stair steppers aren't as popular as the previous three exercise machines, but they can give you a pretty good HIIT workout while sculpting your legs and butt. Be forewarned that it can be difficult to get your heart rate into the right zone with stair stepper routines because your quads may start burning too much to keep going at full speed before you reach the zone you're trying to get into.

There are two common types of steppers. One looks like a moving staircase that you walk or run up and the other has two pedals you apply pressure to in order to simulate walking or running up steps. Either type can be used for HIIT, but the actual first type work the best. Avoid the mini steppers when it comes to HIIT. They aren't durable enough and it's difficult to keep them balanced while sprinting at full speed.

When using a stair stepper, avoid hanging onto the rails for dear life. Release the rails and do your stepping hands-free for a better workout. It's estimated that grabbing onto the rails can curb up to 20% of the calories you'd burn if you weren't holding onto the rail. Pretend you're Rocky Balboa running up the steps of the Philadelphia Museum of Art with nary a handrail in sight. Practice at slower speeds and work your way up to the faster speeds and you'll be ready for anything the stepper can throw at you.

Be aware that steppers can be rough on your joints and are especially problematic for people who have knee and ankle issues. If you have joint problems, skip the stepper and choose a different HIIT routine. Those who are healthy should only do a stair stepper HIIT routine once or twice a week, at most.

Here's a good stair stepper HIIT routine:

Time	Exercise	Exertion (1 - 10)
5 minutes	Warm up. Light resistance. Low speed.	3 to 5
30 seconds	Heavy resistance. Sprinting speed.	8 to 9
1 minute	Light resistance. Moderate speed.	5 to 7
1 minute	Heavy resistance. Sprinting speed.	8 to 9
1 minute	Light resistance. Moderate speed.	5 to 7
Repeat intervals until 20 minutes have passed.		
5 minutes	Cool down. Light resistance. Low speed.	3 to 5

Feel free to play around with the resistance, the speed and the length of your intervals to get you into the right zone.

There's one problem you need to be aware of with stair stepper HIIT and that's the length of time it takes most steppers to switch speeds. There's a few seconds lag time as the machine slows down or ramps up speed, so be sure to factor that in when you're changing speeds. If you're planning on giving it all you've got for a minute, an extra 5 to 8 seconds tacked onto the end of each interval could be the difference between finishing a workout and burning out early.

owing Machine HIIT

When it comes time to hit the machines at the gym for cardio, most people skip the rowing machine. That's too bad because it's one of the only machines that conditions and tones both the upper and lower body while providing the user with an aerobic workout. The rowing machine works a number of major muscle groups, so it's one of the better cardiovascular machines in the gym.

Regardless of your level of fitness, the rowing machine has benefits. A study of elite state-level rowers seeking to compare the results of standard-state training vs. HIIT training on a rowing machine found HIIT to be more effective in reducing body fat and improving overall fitness in comparison to steady-state training. HIIT was also found to improve the amount of adiponectin in the body (11). Low adiponectin levels may be one of the factors that leads to obesity because it plays a role in metabolizing fats (12).

The workout the rowers engaged in was an intense routine that involved eight 2 ½-minute intervals at 90% of their 4-minute maximal power followed by an active recovery period consisting of rowing at 40% of mean four-minute maximal power until the athlete's heart rate dropped back down to 70% (11).

This workout isn't recommended for the average exerciser and instead is designed to push elite athletes to perform at a high level. The average exerciser looking to engage in a HIIT workout will likely find the following workout more than sufficient:

Time	Exercise	Exertion

		(1 - 10)
5 minutes	Warm up. Light resistance.	3 to 5
30 seconds	Heavy resistance. Maximum effort.	8 to 9
1 minute	Light resistance. Moderate effort.	5 to 7
Repeat intervals until 20 minutes have passed.		
5 minutes	Cool down. Light resistance. Low speed.	3 to 5

This routine may not seem like much, but give it a shot and see for yourself how taxing it can be.

Some rowing machines have resistance settings that can be adjusted, while other machines use fans that automatically set the resistance based on how hard you're pulling. If you're using a machine with adjustable resistance, set the resistance as high as you can handle for the high-intensity intervals and push yourself as hard as you can for the full 30 seconds. If the machine adjusts automatically, you'll get a good workout by pulling as hard as you can during the high-intensity intervals and backing off to more gentle pulling for the active recovery periods. If you can easily handle 30 seconds at the intensity you're at, either increase the resistance or increase the length of time of the intervals.

If it's still too easy, try this pyramid routine:

Time	Exercise	Exertion (1 - 10)
5 minutes	Warm up. Light resistance.	3 to 5
30 seconds	Heavy resistance. Maximum effort.	8 to 9
30 seconds	Light resistance. Moderate effort.	5 to 7
45 seconds	Heavy resistance. Maximum effort.	8 to 9
45 seconds	Light resistance. Moderate effort.	5 to 7
1 minute	Heavy resistance. Maximum effort.	8 to 9
1 minute	Light resistance. Moderate effort.	5 to 7
2 minutes	Heavy resistance. Maximum effort.	8 to 9
2 minutes	Light resistance. Moderate effort.	5 to 7
1 minute	Heavy resistance. Maximum effort.	8 to 9
1 minute	Light resistance. Moderate effort.	5 to 7
45 seconds	Heavy resistance. Maximum effort.	8 to 9
45 seconds	Light resistance. Moderate effort.	5 to 7
30 seconds	Heavy resistance. Maximum effort.	8 to 9

30 seconds	Light resistance. Moderate effort.	5 to 7
5 minutes	Cool down. Light resistance. Low speed.	3 to 5

In order to get a full 20+ minute HIIT workout in, cycle through the interval pyramid twice—if you can. Most people will struggle to make it through the pyramid once.

Some rowing machines allow you to set the distance you want to row. You can do pyramids or intervals based on distance instead of time if you'd like. Start at 100 meters on and 100 meters off. Increase the distances for your intervals as you see fit.

If you've got lower back, shoulder or hip issues, the rowing machine probably isn't a good choice for a HIIT routine. Rowing places a lot of stress on all of these areas, so choosing a different workout may help prevent wear and tear on already-damaged areas.

HIIT at Home: Bodyweight Workouts

The beauty of HIIT workouts is they can be done using almost any method of working out you can imagine. Bodyweight workouts are nice because they require no equipment other than your body and somehow still manage to work multiple muscle groups at once.

The bodyweight workouts described in this chapter are perfect for those days when you don't have time to hit the gym and want to get a quick workout in at home or while on the road. All you need is enough space to do jumping jacks, sit ups, push-ups or any of a number of other bodyweight exercises. Some exercises like the bear crawl will require more open space, but you can exclude them from your workout if you have limited space.

Before we get into the routines, let's take a look at the many bodyweight exercises you can do during your bodyweight HIIT routine.

Bench Dips

Difficulty: Moderate.

Best Suited For: Active recovery.

Equipment: Bench (or a sturdy chair).

Muscles Worked: Triceps, Shoulders, Chest.

Here's an exercise that'll build muscle and will torch your triceps if you do it during a HIIT session. You're going to need to be in good shape to do this exercise at a fast enough pace to get your heart rate in the right zone, so it's probably best to use it as an active recovery exercise.

In order to do a bench dip, sit down on a bench and extend your legs out so that they're perpendicular to the bench. Place your feet on another bench or a plyo box that's a foot or two off of the ground. Slide your butt off the bench, and support the full weight of your body with your arms. Slowly lower your body until your butt is a foot or more below the bench and use your triceps to push your body back up until your arms are straight. This is one rep.

Remember, this is HIIT and not a regular workout. You aren't trying to do a certain number of sets or reps. Work at the pace that's right for the type of interval you're doing.

Bodyweight Squats

Difficulty: Easy.

Best Suited For: Active recovery.

Equipment: None.

Muscles Worked: Legs, Glutes, Core.

Your feet should be shoulder-width apart when doing bodyweight squats. Squat as low as you can go and then return to the starting position. It's important to keep your back properly aligned and to make sure your knees don't get in front of your toes.

Jump squats are a variation of bodyweight squats that are a good fit for HIIT routines. With jump squats, instead of slowly lifting yourself back to your starting position, you explosively jump out of the squat. When you land, do so with your legs slightly bent and quickly return to the squatting position.

Lateral Jump

Difficulty: Easy to Moderate.

Best Suited For: High-Intensity Intervals.

Equipment: Weights.

Muscles Worked: Legs, Glutes.

Lateral jumps require that you bound from side-to-side. Push off with one leg and launch your body sideways. As you land, shift your weight to the leg you're landing on. Bend your knee slightly and instantly spring back in the other direction.

For added difficulty, stack a few weights in your jump path. Leap over the weights with each lateral jump. Be very careful not to catch your leg or feet on the weights as you jump. Trust me when I say it'll leave a mark and may put you out of commission for some time.

Bear Crawl

Difficulty: Moderate.

Best Suited For: High-Intensity Intervals.

Equipment: None.

Muscles Worked: Full body.

Anyone who played football in high school probably did enough of this exercise to last them a lifetime. In order to bear crawl, you're going to need 20 to 30 yards of unimpeded open space, preferably on a soft surface like grass or turf. Run along the ground on all fours, using both your arms and legs to propel your body. When done right, it looks similar to a bear running.

This workout is technically a full-body workout, but it tends to put a heavier strain on your upper body. When done right during a HIIT session, bear crawls will leave your upper body quivering and begging for mercy

Burpees

Difficulty: Hard.

Best Suited For: High-Intensity Intervals.

Equipment: Dumbbells (optional).

Muscles Worked: Full body.

Also known as squat thrusts, burpees are one of the most hated and beloved of all bodyweight exercises. Novice exercisers tend to hate burpees because of their difficulty, while veterans love them because they know they're working their entire body with each and every burpee they do.

Burpees should be part of your workout routine, regardless of what sort of workouts you're doing. They're great for burning calories, gaining strength, conditioning your body and they can be added to pretty much any workout.

Here are the directions for doing a proper burpee:

1. Stand straight up and down with your feet shoulder-width apart.
2. Lower yourself into a squatting position and place your hand on the floor, slightly ahead of your body.
3. Jump back with your feet so that your body is in push-up position.
4. Do a push-up.
5. Jump your feet back to their original squat position.

6. Push hard as you come out of the squat, forcing your body to jump into the air.
7. Clap your hands over your head as you reach the peak of the jump.
8. Repeat until your body is begging for mercy.

If you're looking for a more difficult version of burpees, do them while holding light dumbbells during the jumping portion of the burpee. You can either set the weights off to either side of your body during the push-ups or you can really amp up the difficulty by holding onto the dumbbells while doing the push-ups, too.

Butt Kickers

Difficulty: Easy.

Best Suited For: Can be used for Active recovery or High-Intensity Intervals. Vary the pace accordingly.

Equipment: None.

Muscles Worked: Legs, Glutes.

Stand straight up and down with your feet resting at approximately hip-width apart. Lift one leg at a time, kicking yourself in the butt with the heel of your shoe. Run as fast as you can, lightly tapping your butt with each heel every time you lift each of your legs.

Once you've got the butt kickers mastered, try jumping butt kickers. With these, you jump in the air and kick yourself in the butt with both feet at once. Try alternating, left foot, right foot, jump, left foot, right foot jump for an intense workout that'll leave you gasping for breath.

High Knees

Difficulty: Easy.

Best Suited For: Can be used for Active recovery or High-Intensity Intervals. Vary the pace accordingly.

Equipment: None.

Muscles Worked: Legs, Glutes, Core.

High knees are similar to marching in place at high speed. Stand with your feet hip-width apart. Raise one knee up until it's even with your hip. Now switch knees and run in place, lifting each knee to hip-height as you run.

This exercise can be one of your core exercises for bodyweight HIIT workouts. High knees can be used for high-intensity intervals if you do them at a fast pace or you can slow down and do them at a slower pace during active recovery periods.

Jumping

Difficulty: Easy.

Best Suited For: Can be used for Active recovery or High-Intensity Intervals. Vary the pace accordingly.

Equipment: Plyo box (optional) or jump rope (optional).

Muscles Worked: Legs, Glutes.

Everybody knows how to jump, although it may have been a while since some of us have had both feet off the ground. **Explosive jumping** is the act of squatting low and exploding into a jump that's as far off the ground as you can get. Be sure to land with your knees slightly bent and instantly squat down for your next jump. Each jump should be as explosive as you're capable of.

If you're looking to step up the difficulty, try jumping with your arms held straight out in front of you or crossed over your chest. You can also try jumping onto a platform or a plyo box, if you have one available. Plyo boxes are designed for box jumps and should be sturdy enough to hold your weight.

Jumping rope is a great exercise for high-intensity intervals. It'll get your heart rate up fast and keep it high through the interval, as long as you're able to time your jumps right and keep jumping at a high rate of speed.

Jumping Jacks

Difficulty: Easy.

Best Suited For: Can be used for Active recovery or High-Intensity Intervals. Vary the pace accordingly.

Equipment: None.

Muscles Worked: Legs, Glutes.

Stand in an erect position, with your feet close together and your arms hanging at your side. Jump in the air. While in the air, raise your arms and open up your feet to beyond shoulder width. Land in this position. Jump in the air again and return to the starting position with your feet close together and your arms at your sides.

Jumping jacks work your calves, hip adductors, shoulders and core. Speed them up and they're a great cardio exercise. Slow them down and you can do them during active recovery periods as well.

Lunges

Difficulty: Easy.

Best Suited For: Active recovery.

Equipment: Barbell or dumbbells.

Muscles Worked: Legs, Glutes.

Stand tall with your feet together. Step out with your right foot and slowly lower your body until your right knee is bent at least 90 degrees and your thigh is parallel to the ground. Return to the starting position and step out with your left foot and do the same thing.

This exercise can be made harder by holding a barbell on your shoulders or holding dumbbells in each of your hands and letting them hang by your side while you do the lunges. For a really brutal workout, hold a heavy weight plate out in front of you and twist from side to side with your arms fully extended after each rep.

Mountain Climbers

Difficulty: Easy to Moderate.

Best Suited For: Can be used for Active recovery or High-Intensity Intervals. Vary the pace accordingly.

Equipment: None.

Muscles Worked: Legs, Core.

Position yourself like you've just done a push-up and are in the arms extended position. Move your right leg forward until the knee is almost touching your right elbow and place your foot flat on the ground. Rapidly switch leg positions. After the switch, your left leg should be forward and your right leg will be extended behind you. This is one rep.

Continue jumping and switching legs until you're in the right zone for the type of interval you're doing. This is a good exercise for either active recovery or high-intensity intervals because you can easily dictate the pace at which you do mountain climbers.

Plank

Difficulty: Moderate to Hard.

Best Suited For: Depends on what kind of shape you're in.

Equipment: None.

Muscles Worked: Abs, Core.

Lay flat on the floor on your stomach with your legs extended out behind you. Lying prone, lift yourself up and support your body weight on your toes and your forearms. Hold this position for as long as possible. If you've never planked before, you're in for a special treat. No exercise works your body quite in the same way a long plank does. If you can hold it for a minute, you're doing pretty good.

Up the difficulty by raising an arm or a leg off the ground. Experts can raise one arm and one leg.

The type of interval planking is best suited for depends on what kind of shape you're in. If you're out of shape, planking may be strenuous enough to get your heart rate into the right zone for high-intensity intervals. If you're in good shape, it's best used as an active recovery exercise.

Pull-Ups

Difficulty: Hard.

Best Suited For: High-Intensity Intervals.

Equipment: Bar, bands or box (optional).

Muscles Worked: Back, Shoulders, Arms.

You're going to need to be in prime shape if you plan on incorporating pull-ups into your HIIT routine. This is one of the most taxing bodyweight exercises there is and most people outside of the fitness world are lucky to be able to do a single pull-up.

If you're like most people and can only do a pull-up or two before you're unable to continue, you can still incorporate pull-ups into your routine with a little ingenuity. You can stand on a box or a bench and use it to support some of your weight while you do the pull-ups. This allows you to adjust the amount of weight you're lifting with each and every pull-up. Ideally, you'll barely be able to finish each one. Alternatively, you can use bands to support some of your weight.

Pull-ups are done with your hands facing away from your body. Chin-ups can also be part of your routine and are done with the palms of your hand facing your body. A pull-up or chin-up isn't complete until the entire head has been lifted above the bar. Some gyms have pull-up assist machines that will help novices complete pull-ups.

Push-Ups

Difficulty: Moderate.

Best Suited For: High-Intensity Intervals.

Equipment: None.

Muscles Worked: Upper body, Core.

Push-ups are a bodyweight exercise designed to strengthen the core and the upper body. They work out the arms, chest, shoulders, abs, triceps, neck and back all at the same time.

Diamond push-ups are done with the hands close together, with the thumb and index finger forming a diamond shape. The closer your hands are together, the more focus there is on the triceps. Consequentially, the further apart your hands are, the better the workout is for your chest and back. Push-ups can be done on an incline, in order to focus on the chest and core muscles, or on a decline, which focuses the effort on the legs, back and the core.

Elite athletes may want to do one-arm push-ups. Using only one arm at a time works one side of the chest and the triceps on one side individually, forcing the core to work overtime to keep the body balanced. One-armed push-ups are difficult and are best left to the experienced exercisers.

Sit-Ups

Difficulty: Easy to Moderate.

Best Suited For: High-Intensity Intervals.

Equipment: None.

Muscles Worked: Abdominal, Core.

In order to do sit-ups during a HIIT session, you're going to have to be able to do enough sit-ups to get your heart rate into the right zone. If you're only able to do a handful of sit-ups before you're in too much pain to continue, choose different exercises for HIIT until you're in better shape. Try incorporating sit-ups into your non-HIIT routines until you're able to do enough of them to add them to your high-intensity interval training sessions.

Crunches are a variation of the sit-up in which you only partially lift your body. They may be more appropriate for the amateur to moderate athlete. Don't underestimate the power of crunches. They'll still give you a pretty good workout. Try doing them with your hands extended out in front of your body or with your fingers interlocked behind your head.

Stair Climb

Difficulty: Moderate to Hard.

Best Suited For: Can be used for Active recovery or High-Intensity Intervals. Vary the pace accordingly.

Equipment: Weights (optional).

Muscles Worked: Legs, Glutes.

Running up and down stairs will get your heart rate in the right zone in a hurry. It'll also help you build up your leg muscles and your endurance. You get the added bonus of stronger leg bones because climbing stairs causes the muscles in your legs to pull on the bones, making them stronger and denser.

Stair climbs can be done anywhere there's stairs that aren't too crowded to run up and down. Keep a watchful eye out for local places that have a lot of wide-open stairs. High school and college sports stadiums usually have a lot of stairs, as do high-rise and apartment buildings, although gaining access to them may be problematic. When all else fails, you may be able to hit the stairs at home if you have a 2- or 3-story house.

Try adding weights to your stair climbs to get a better workout. You can carry dumbbells or strap a weight vest on and start climbing.

Wall Sit

Difficulty: Easy to Moderate.

Best Suited For: Active recovery.

Equipment: Weights (optional).

Muscles Worked: Legs, Glutes, Back.

Place your back against a wall. Slide down the wall until your thighs are parallel to the ground. It should look like you're trying to sit on an invisible chair.

Wall sits aren't intense enough to get your heart rate into the right zone for the high-intensity intervals, but they work well as an active recovery exercise. If you want to work harder, try doing bicep curls with dumbbells while in the sitting position.

Bodyweight HIIT Routines

Designing your own bodyweight HIIT routines is easy. All you have to do is pick a handful of bodyweight exercises you'd like to include in your routine and decide on an interval length. It helps to remmeber the goal of HIIT is to reach maximum exertion on each interval. Choose bodyweight exercises that will push you to the limit for the high-intensity intervals. Save the easier exercises for the active recovery periods.

The rest of this section covers a variety of bodyweight HIIT routines designed to leave you dripping sweat and sucking for breath by the time they're complete.

Baby Steps

If you're out of shape, you aren't going to jump right into a 20-minute HIIT routine and knock it out of the park. You're probably going to burn out somewhere between 5 and 10 minutes into the workout. This is normal and we all went through it at one point of time. The first time I tried a HIIT routine, I was out of breath before the warm-up session was complete.

I wish I would have had a workout tailored to beginners when I first started. If you've spent a good portion of your life behind a desk and your idea of exercise is getting up to walk to the kitchen, even this routine is going to be tough. Finish what you can and push yourself to go a little further every time you work out.

It's surprising what you can accomplish in a half hour three or four days a week, but you've got to stick with it. If you work out once and then wait a couple weeks between HIIT sessions, you're going to be starting over again every time you exercise. You won't make much by way of gains when your sessions are sporadic.

Here's the Baby Steps workout, designed to get your feet wet:

Time/Distance	Exercise	Exertion (1 - 10)
2 minutes	Warm up. Light jogging in place.	3 to 5
15 seconds	Full-speed jumping jacks.	8 to 9
45 seconds	Light jogging in place.	5 to 7

15 seconds	Butt kickers. As fast as you can.	8 to 9
45 seconds	Light jogging in place.	5 to 7
15 seconds	High knees. As fast as you can.	8 to 9
45 seconds	Light jogging in place.	5 to 7
15 seconds	Mountain climbers. As fast as you can.	8 to 9
45 seconds	Light jogging in place.	5 to 7
15 seconds	Burpees.	8 to 9
45 seconds	Light jogging in place.	5 to 7
Repeat intervals one more time, if you can.		
2 minutes	Cool down. Light jogging in place.	3 to 5

Once you're able to do this routine and can cycle through the intervals twice, up the time of the high-intensity intervals to 30 seconds. Try to leave the active recovery periods at 45 seconds, but you can extend them to a minute, if need be. Depending on what kind of shape you're in, it could take weeks or even months before you're ready to add time to the intervals. Everyone is different, so don't get frustrated. Stick with it and you'll slowly but surely improve.

Slowly increase your high-intensity interval times until they're at a minute and the active recovery times are at a minute. Once you're able to do that, you'll be ready to try some of the other routines in this chapter and the rest of the book. Go slow and only do what you're capable of. It's going to be hard, but shouldn't be so hard you end up hurting yourself.

Give your body time to adjust to the pounding it's going to take in the first couple weeks and you'll be much better off.

The Bear Blaster

The Bear Blaster combines two exercises to create a routine that's going to absolutely torch your triceps and upper body. It requires that you're able to bear crawl in multiple directions, going backward, forward and laterally.

Here's the workout:

Time/Distance	Exercise	Exertion (1 - 10)
5 minutes	Warm up. Light jogging or light bodyweight exercises.	3 to 5
Not applicable	30- to 50-yard bear crawl forward at full speed.	8 to 9
Not applicable	10 push-ups. Followed by light jogging in place until your heart rate reaches the right zone.	5 to 7
Not applicable	20- to 30-yard lateral bear crawl at full speed.	8 to 9
Not applicable	10 push-ups. Followed by light jogging in place until your heart rate reaches the right zone.	5 to 7
Not applicable	30- to 50-yard bear crawl backward at full speed.	8 to 9
Not applicable	10 push-ups. Followed by light jogging in place until your heart rate reaches the right zone.	5 to 7
Not applicable	20- to 30-yard lateral bear	8 to 9

	crawl at full speed. Return to starting position.	
Not applicable	10 push-ups. Followed by light jogging in place until your heart rate reaches the right zone.	5 to 7
Repeat intervals until 20 minutes have passed.		
5 minutes	Light jogging or light bodyweight exercises.	3 to 5

When doing this routine, the bear crawls should be done in the shape of a rectangle, so that you crawl forward, laterally, backwards and then laterally in the opposite direction to return to your starting position.

Burp-Ups

The name of this routine may be a little off-putting, but combining burpees with sit-ups, push-ups and pull-ups sets this workout apart from the rest in that it's a full-body workout on steroids. OK, bad analogy, but it's a great workout nonetheless.

Time/Distance	Exercise	Exertion (1 - 10)
5 minutes	Warm up. Moderate-speed butt kickers, followed by high knees.	3 to 5
45 seconds	Fast-paced burpees.	8 to 9
1 minute	Moderate-paced sit-ups.	5 to 7
45 seconds	Fast-paced burpees.	8 to 9
1 minute	Moderate-paced pull-ups. Use assist, if necessary.	5 to 7
45 seconds	Fast-paced burpees.	8 to 9
1 minute	Moderate-paced push-ups. Rest for a few seconds at the top of each push-up, if necessary.	5 to 7
Repeat intervals until 20 minutes have passed.		
5 minutes	Cool down. Moderate-speed butt kickers, followed by high knees.	3 to 5

Climbing Everest

This routine is called Climbing Everest because it combines mountain climbers with burpees and will leave you feeling like you've just attempted to climb Mount Everest after just a few intervals.

Here's the workout:

Time/Distance	Exercise	Exertion (1 - 10)
5 minutes	Warm up. Slow to moderate speed mountain climbers for a couple minutes, followed by jogging in place.	3 to 5
30 seconds	Full-intensity burpees. Do them as fast as you can.	8 to 9
1 minute	Moderate speed mountain climbers.	5 to 7
Repeat intervals until 20 minutes have passed.		
5 minutes	Cool down. Slow to moderate speed mountain climbers for a couple minutes, followed by jogging in place.	3 to 5

Jump 'N Sit

Combine lateral jumps, jumping jacks and wall sits and what do you get? A leg and core workout that'll destroy your legs while helping kick your body into afterburn mode for days on end.

Here's the Jump 'N Sit routine:

Time/Distance	Exercise	Exertion (1 - 10)
5 minutes	Warm up. Light to moderate speed lateral jumps and jumping jacks.	3 to 5
30 seconds	Full-speed lateral jumps.	8 to 9
30 seconds	Wall sit.	5 to 7
45 seconds	Full-speed jumping jacks.	8 to 9
45 seconds	Wall sit.	5 to 7
Repeat intervals until 20 minutes have passed.		
5 minutes	Cool down. Light to moderate speed lateral jumps and jumping jacks.	3 to 5

Stairway to Heaven

The best way to do HIIT while climbing stairs will depend on how many stairs there are at the place you plan on working out. Ideally, you'll have somewhere to work out with enough stairs to climb to where you're exhausted once you get to the top of the flight. If the flight of stairs is too long, stop halfway up and slowly jog back down.

Here's a sample HIIT routine that incorporates stairs to make sure you get a good workout:

Time/Distance	Exercise	Exertion (1 - 10)
5 minutes	Warm up. Light jogging or light bodyweight exercises.	3 to 5
Not applicable	Start at the bottom of the stairs. Run full speed up the stairs.	8 to 9
Not applicable	Lightly jog back down to the bottom of the stairs.	5 to 7
Repeat intervals until 20 minutes have passed.		
5 minutes	Light jogging or light bodyweight exercises.	3 to 5

The key to getting a good HIIT stairway routine in is to go all-out all the way up the stairs and then give yourself time to recover on your way back down. At my local high school stadium, there's a long flight of stairs that divides the bleachers in half. At the top of these stairs is a pathway that loops around and back down to the field. My HIIT routine consists of a series of sprints up the stairs and light jogs down the pathway and back around to the bottom of the stairs.

Walk the Plank

Walk the Plank is designed for people who are in great shape because it requires being able to hold a plank for 45 seconds to a minute. Your entire body is going to get a workout with this routine:

Time/Distance	Exercise	Exertion (1 - 10)
5 minutes	Warm up. Light to moderate high knees.	3 to 5
30 seconds	Full-speed high knees.	8 to 9
30 seconds	Plank. If heart rate isn't low enough after plank, jog in place until it reaches the right zone.	5 to 7
45 seconds	Full-speed butt kickers.	8 to 9
45 seconds	Plank. If heart rate isn't low enough after plank, jog in place until it reaches the right zone.	5 to 7
1 minute	Full-speed butt kickers.	8 to 9
1 minute	Plank. If heart rate isn't low enough after plank, jog in place until it reaches the right zone.	5 to 7
Repeat intervals until 20 minutes have passed.		
5 minutes	Cool down. Light to	3 to 5

	moderate high knees.	

The Ultimate Workout

This HIIT routine isn't for the faint of heart. It isn't so much a workout, as it's a leg-crushing, arm-pounding, core-pummeling test of your athletic ability.

Enough with the build-up; here's the workout:

Time/Distance	Exercise	Exertion (1 - 10)
3 minutes	Warm up. Light- to moderate-speed jumping jacks.	3 to 5
1 minute	Full-speed forward bear crawl.	8 to 9
1 minute	Light- to moderate -speed bench dips.	5 to 7
1 minute	Full-speed butt kickers.	8 to 9
1 minute	Moderate-speed high knees.	5 to 7
1 minute	Burpees.	8 to 9
1 minute	Plank.	5 to 7
1 minute	Full-speed lateral jump.	8 to 9
1 minute	Sit-ups.	5 to 7
1 minute	Full-speed mountain climbers.	8 to 9
1 minute	Wall sit.	5 to 7
1 minute	Full-speed reverse bear crawl.	8 to 9
1 minute	Light- to moderate -speed	5 to 7

	bench dips.	
1 minute	Full-speed butt kickers.	8 to 9
1 minute	Moderate-speed high knees.	5 to 7
1 minute	Burpees.	8 to 9
1 minute	Plank.	5 to 7
1 minute	Full-speed lateral jump.	8 to 9
1 minute	Sit-ups.	5 to 7
1 minute	Full-speed mountain climbers.	8 to 9
1 minute	Wall sit.	5 to 7
3 minutes	Warm up. Light- to moderate-speed jumping jacks.	3 to 5

If you aren't completely exhausted by the time this routine is finished, there's something seriously wrong with you.

Design Your Own Bodyweight HIIT Routine

It's relatively easy to design your own bodyweight HIIT routines. All you need to do is pair good high-intensity interval exercises with good active recovery exercises that will allow your heart rate to recover enough to get ready for the next intense interval.

A standard bodyweight HIIT routine could follow this format:

Time/Distance	Exercise	Exertion (1 - 10)
5 minutes	Warm up. Slow- to moderate-speed active recovery exercise.	3 to 5
30 seconds to 1 minute	Full-intensity exercise.	8 to 9
30 seconds to 2 minutes	Active recovery exercise done at moderate speed.	5 to 7
Repeat intervals until 20 minutes have passed.		
5 minutes	Slow- to moderate-speed active recovery exercise.	3 to 5

Bodyweight HIIT routines can also be designed as pyramid routines, which will follow the following template:

Time/Distance	Exercise	Exertion (1 - 10)

5 minutes	Warm up. Slow- to moderate-speed active recovery exercise.	3 to 5
30 seconds	Full-intensity exercise.	8 to 9
30 seconds	Active recovery exercise done at moderate speed.	5 to 7
45 seconds	Full-intensity exercise.	8 to 9
45 seconds	Active recovery exercise done at moderate speed.	5 to 7
1 minute	Full-intensity exercise.	8 to 9
1 minute	Active recovery exercise done at moderate speed.	5 to 7
1 minute	Full-intensity exercise.	8 to 9
1 minute	Active recovery exercise done at moderate speed.	5 to 7
45 seconds	Full-intensity exercise.	8 to 9
45 seconds	Active recovery exercise done at moderate speed.	5 to 7
30 seconds	Full-intensity exercise.	8 to 9
30 seconds	Active recovery exercise done at moderate speed.	5 to 7
Repeat the pyramid a second time, if you're able to.		
5 minutes	Slow- to moderate-speed active recovery exercise.	3 to 5

You can mix-and-match the exercises done in the routines or you can pick a couple exercises and stick with them all the way through the entire routine. It's your call.

Tabata Training: The 4-Minute Workout

Would you believe me if I said you could get in shape using a workout known as a Tabata workout that takes just 4 minutes of your time.

The workout was designed by a Japanese Olympic Speed Skating Team Coach who created an intense 4-minute workout for his athletes. The workout consisted of 20 seconds of intense cycling followed by 10 seconds of rest repeated for 8 rounds, for a grand total of 4 minutes. One of his assistant coaches tested the program and found the athletes participating in it had gained almost 30% in anaerobic capacity and had realized a 14% gain in their VO2 max. The gains were significantly higher in the Tabata group than in a control group that was doing hour-long training sessions 5 days a week (13).

Since this discovery, Tabata training has evolved to include other exercise routines that follow a 20-second on/10-second off format. It can be done with pretty much any type of exercise, including bodyweight exercises, aerobic exercises, sprinting and can be adapted to work on a number of exercise machines.

If you're thinking Tabata sounds a lot like a quick HIIT session, you're right, but there are a handful of differences. For one, the average HIIT session lasts 20 minutes—30 to 40 if you factor in warm-ups—while a normal Tabata session lasts a total of 4 minutes. Another key difference between Tabata and normal HIIT sessions are the rest periods used in Tabata sessions are actual rest periods where no exercises are done. HIIT rest periods are active recovery periods, where light to moderate exercise is done.

The basic characteristics of a Tabata session are as follows:

The entire workout is 4 minutes long. You'll see workouts online and even in books claiming to be Tabata workouts that are 20 minutes or longer. These workouts are usually HIIT routines and they'll get you in shape, but they aren't technically Tabata. True Tabata routines only last 4 minutes.

20 seconds on, 10 seconds off. The high-intensity intervals last for 20 seconds and are punctuated by 10-second rest periods. The high-intensity intervals should be done at as fast a pace as you can manage while still maintaining good form. The 10-second rest periods are total rest. No exercise is done during these periods.

8 rounds. Each round of intervals lasts a total of 30 seconds and the intervals are repeated 8 times, creating a workout that meets the Tabata requirement of being 4 minutes long.

It's intense. Each of the eight 20-second intervals should be as intense as you can make them while still maintaining good form. The idea is to achieve the maximum number of reps you during the 20-second interval. Constantly trying to improve your max reps will ensure you're pushing as hard as you can. You're only going to be doing them for 20 seconds, so push hard. Don't leave anything in your reserves.

The original Tabata routine only used one exercise. Here is an example of a simple Tabata routine that does the same:

Time/Distance	Exercise	Exertion (1 - 10)
20 seconds	Full-speed sprinting.	8 to 9
10 seconds	Rest.	1
Repeat the intervals 8 times, for a total workout lasting 4 minutes.		

You can combine exercises to create a variation of the Tabata routine that involves a variety of exercises. This routine calls for 2 sets of 4 different exercises:

Time/Distance	Exercise	Exertion (1 - 10)
20 seconds	Burpees.	8 to 9
10 seconds	Rest.	1
20 seconds	Bodyweight squats.	8 to 9
10 seconds	Rest.	1
20 seconds	Overhead slam (with medicine ball).	8 to 9
10 seconds	Rest.	1
20 seconds	Push-ups.	8 to 9
10 seconds	Rest.	1

Repeat intervals a second time.

The following routine calls for 8 different exercises in a single Tabata routine:

Time/Distance	Exercise	Exertion (1 - 10)
20 seconds	Jumping jacks.	8 to 9
10 seconds	Rest.	1
20 seconds	Burpees.	8 to 9
10 seconds	Rest.	1
20 seconds	Sit-ups.	8 to 9
10 seconds	Rest.	1
20 seconds	Push-ups.	8 to 9
10 seconds	Rest.	1
20 seconds	Jump rope.	8 to 9
10 seconds	Rest.	1
20 seconds	Mountain climbers.	8 to 9
10 seconds	Rest.	1
20 seconds	Bear crawl.	8 to 9
10 seconds	Rest.	1
20 seconds	Full-speed sprinting.	8 to 9
10 seconds	Rest.	1

Pick and choose the exercises you want to do based on what muscle group(s) you want to work on that day. For example, if you're planning on working on your legs, choose exercises like squats, burpees, butt kickers and lunges. If you're working on your abs, be sure to include planking and a variety of sit-ups. Arm days can include weight training exercises like curls and body weight exercises like bench dips, triangle push-ups and pull-ups.

The Tabata HIIT Routine

Depending on the shape you're in, you may leave a Tabata 4-minute session feeling like you really didn't get much accomplished. It's a great workout for beginners and those who are new to HIIT, because it allows you to give 100% for 4 minutes, which is about as short a workout as you're going to find.

While Tabata has been shown to have good results with elite athletes, you may find yourself wanting more at some point. Once you're

I designed this Tabata HIIT routine to push you to the limit and beyond. It takes a standard 4-minute Tabata session and multiplies it by 5 to create a 20-minute workout that's a combination of both HIIT and Tabata. To top things off, the 10-second rest periods typical of Tabata have been replaced by 10 seconds of the same exercise you just did in the high-intensity interval, but at a slower pace.

This is the basic template for the Tabata HIIT routine. You can use this template to design your own Tabata HIIT workouts:

Time/Distance	Exercise	Exertion (1 - 10)
20 seconds	High-intensity exercise.	8 to 9
10 seconds	Same exercise, but at a slower pace.	5 to 7
Repeat 8 times for a total of 4 minutes.		

20 seconds	High-intensity exercise.	8 to 9
10 seconds	Same exercise, but at a slower pace.	5 to 7

Repeat 8 times for a total of 4 minutes.

20 seconds	High-intensity exercise.	8 to 9
10 seconds	Same exercise, but at a slower pace.	5 to 7

Repeat 8 times for a total of 4 minutes.

20 seconds	High-intensity exercise.	8 to 9
10 seconds	Same exercise, but at a slower pace.	5 to 7

Repeat 8 times for a total of 4 minutes.

20 seconds	High-intensity exercise.	8 to 9
10 seconds	Same exercise, but at a slower pace.	5 to 7

Repeat 8 times for a total of 4 minutes.

This workout is one of the most difficult workouts in the book, so make sure you're in prime physical shape before attempting it. A variation of this exercise calls for 30-second to 1-minute rest periods between each of the Tabata sessions and looks something like this:

Time/Distance	Exercise	Exertion (1 - 10)
20 seconds	High-intensity exercise.	8 to 9
10 seconds	Same exercise, but at a slower pace.	5 to 7
Repeat 8 times for a total of 4 minutes.		
Rest for 30 seconds to 1 minute.		
20 seconds	High-intensity exercise.	8 to 9
10 seconds	Same exercise, but at a slower pace.	5 to 7
Repeat 8 times for a total of 4 minutes.		
Rest for 30 seconds to 1 minute.		
20 seconds	High-intensity exercise.	8 to 9

10 seconds	Same exercise, but at a slower pace.	5 to 7

Repeat 8 times for a total of 4 minutes.

Rest for 30 seconds to 1 minute.

20 seconds	High-intensity exercise.	8 to 9
10 seconds	Same exercise, but at a slower pace.	5 to 7

Repeat 8 times for a total of 4 minutes.

Rest for 30 seconds to 1 minute.

20 seconds	High-intensity exercise.	8 to 9
10 seconds	Same exercise, but at a slower pace.	5 to 7

Repeat 8 times for a total of 4 minutes.

This workout will still be tiring, but should be a little more manageable than the original Tabata HIIT routine.

You can also make things easier by cutting the workout down to 10 minutes instead of a full 20 until you get used to it.

Combine HIIT with Weight Training for Great Results

If you incorporate weight training into your workout regimen, try adding HIIT or Tabata training sessions to your weight training routines to trim fat and help tone your muscles. I sometimes add a couple Tabata sessions to my workout days and then do full HIIT routines once or twice a week on my days off.

Other times, I incorporate HIIT into my weight training sessions by creating a weight training routine that adds light cardio to intervals of weight lifting. Instead of counting reps during these workouts, I lift for a certain amount of time. Choose weights that will allow you to just barely make it to the end of the interval. It makes for a difficult workout, especially when the lactic acid really starts to build up near the end of the routine.

If you hit a point during an interval where your muscles start to fail, stop just long enough to where you can lift again and get back at it. If you need to, take a 15- to 30-second breather at the end of each interval set.

Here's a template you can use to create your own HIIT weight training routine:

Time/Distance	Exercise	Exertion (1 - 10)
1 minute	Warm up. Light to moderate cardio.	3 to 5
30 seconds	Warm up. Light to	8 to 9

	moderate lifting exercise.	
30 seconds	Heavy lifting exercise. Perform as many lifts as you can in 30 seconds.	8 to 9
15 seconds	Light cardio.	5 to 7
Repeat intervals until 20 minutes have passed.		

You could also do the opposite of what's done in the previous workout, opting to do intense cardio during the high-intensity intervals followed by light lifting sessions during the active recovery periods. This is what the alternate workout would look like:

Time/Distance	Exercise	Exertion (1 - 10)
1 minute	Warm up. Light to moderate cardio.	3 to 5
30 seconds	Warm up. Light to moderate lifting exercise.	8 to 9
30 seconds	Intense cardio.	8 to 9
15 seconds	Light lifting exercise.	5 to 7
Repeat intervals until 20 minutes have passed.		

The exercises you choose will determine the muscle groups you work in that session. You can opt to concentrate on one muscle group and really hit it hard or you can work different muscle groups to go for a full body routine.

HIIT Tips

The following tips can be used to help ensure you get the most from your workouts while staying safe:

Always warm up. HIIT is intense and can be hard on your body. There's no reason to compound the chance of injury by failing to properly warm up. Light cardio is a good choice for warming up because it gets you moving and begins to elevate your heart rate.

Make sure you choose the right weight. When doing exercises that incorporate weights, choosing the right weight is critical. While you may feel inclined to choose the heaviest weight you can lift, this isn't a good choice because you're going to be doing a lot of reps. You want to choose the heaviest weight you can use to safely perform reps while maintaining good posture. There's a fine line between safe heavy lifting and serious injury. It's up to you to ensure you don't cross it.

Bring it! Push hard during the intense intervals. High-intensity intervals are supposed to be intense. You should be dripping sweat and your heart should be pounding by the time you finish an interval. If not, you probably aren't pushing hard enough.

Make sure you're healthy enough to do HIIT. This type of workout isn't for everyone. If you have health problems, check with your doctor to see if HIIT is a good fit. Even if you don't have health problems, it's a good idea to get a check-up and tell your doctor what you're planning on doing. If you're out of shape, HIIT is going to be extremely tough. There are people who start their fitness journey with HIIT and stick it out, but these people are few and far between. Many beginners would be better served getting in halfway decent shape before trying HIIT.

Keep the intervals short. Most people have a tough time giving everything they've got for 30 seconds. Some athletes can push hard for a minute and elite athletes are able to push for 2 minutes or more. If you're doing intervals that are longer than 2 minutes, you probably aren't doing HIIT. 20-second intervals are the minimum interval length you should be doing.

Mix it up. Don't get stuck on a single workout routine. Your body will get used to doing the same thing over and over and over again. Instead, use different exercise machines and bodyweight workouts to switch things up. Keep your body guessing and you'll be less likely to fall into a rut. You'll also be less likely to burn out and fall victim to repetitive motion injuries.

Don't overdo it. Three HIIT routines a week are all most people should do. Experienced exercisers can push it up to 4 workouts a week. Never do HIIT routines on back-to-back days. Give yourself at least one day between HIIT workouts in order to allow time for your body to recover.

Listen to your body. HIIT sessions are intense. They can take a toll on your body, especially when combined with other types of exercise and/or lifting. If you're extremely sore or have a nagging pain that just won't go away, it may be a good idea to forget about HIIT until your body has had a chance to heal. You don't want to suffer an injury that'll sideline you for weeks or even months. Most injuries come about as a result of people ignoring early indicators that there's a problem. Small problems can become large problems in a hurry if they're ignored.

Closing Thoughts

High-intensity interval training is a great way to lose weight while improving your muscle tone and overall fitness, but you're only going to get out of it what you're willing to put into it. While the workout routines are shorter than the average workout routine, they definitely aren't easy. You have to be willing to pour every last ounce of energy and willpower you have in you into your workout in order to get the results you're looking for.

The appeal of HIIT workouts to some people is the fact that they are much shorter than the average steady-state cardio session. HIIT sessions usually take less than a half hour, while steady-state cardio sessions take 45 minutes to an hour or longer. For some, an hour of cardio is tantamount to torture. Just because HIIT sessions are shorter in duration, don't assume they're going to be easier. If anything, they're harder than steady-state cardio when done right.

Leaving it all in the gym or on the track or in your living room—or wherever else it may be that you're working out—will get you the results you're looking for. Failure to drive your heart rate into the right zone will result in less than stellar gains.

When done right, HIIT gives you more bang for your buck than pretty much any other workout routine in existence. It's a great way to lose weight while building or maintaining muscle mass and will torch fat off your body.

Give HIIT a shot and see if it's right for you. Get strong. Get fit. Get HIIT.

Works Cited

1. *Impact of exercise intensity on body fatness and skeletal muscle metabolism.* **Angelo Tremblay, Jean-Aime Simoneau, Claude Bouchard.** 7, s.l. : Metabolism, 1994, Vol. 43, pp. 814-818.

2. *Effect of 2 weeks of sprint interval training on health-related outcomes in sedentary overweight/obese men.* **Laura J. Whyte, Jason M.R. Gill, Andrew J. Cathcart.** 1, s.l. : Metabolism, 2010, Vol. 24, pp. 153 - 161.

3. *Lipid metabolism in young men after acute resistance exercise at two different intensities.* **S. Hill, M.A. Bermingham, P.K. Knight.** 4, s.l. : Journal of Science and Medicine in Sport, 2005, Vol. 8, pp. 441- 445.

4. *The effects of high-intensity intermittent exercise training on fat loss and fasting insulin levels of young women.* **E G Trapp, D J Chisholm, J Freund, S H Boutcher.** 4, s.l. : Int J Obes (Lond), 2008, Vol. 32, pp. 684 - 691.

5. *Uniqueness of interval and continuous training at the same maintained exercise intensity.* **Gorostiaga EM, Walter CB, Foster C, Hickson RC.** 2, s.l. : Eur J Appl Physiol Occup Physiol, 1991, Vol. 63, pp. 101 - 107.

6. *A Comparison of the Effects of Interval Training vs. Continuous Training on Weight Loss and Body Composition in Obese Pre-Menopausal Women.* **King, Jeffrey Warren.** s.l. : Digital Commons @ East Tennessee State University, 2001.

7. *Run sprint interval training improves aerobic performance but not maximal cardiac output.* **Macpherson RE, Hazell TJ, Olver TD, Paterson DH, Lemon PW.** 1, Jan 2011, Med Sci Sports Exercise, Vol. 43, pp. 115 - 122.

8. *Hormonal and inflammatory responses to different types of sprint interval training.* **Meckel Y, Nemet D, Bar-Sela S, Radom-Aizik S, Cooper DM, Sagiv M, Eliakim A.** 8, Aug 2011, J Strength Cond Res, Vol. 25, pp. 2161 - 2169.

9. *Physiological and performance changes from the addition of a sprint interval program to wrestling training.* **Farzad B, Gharakhanlou R, Agha-Alinejad H, Curby DG, Bayati M, Bahraminejad M, Mäestu J.** 9, Sep 2011, J Strength Cond Res, Vol. 25, pp. 2392 - 2399.

10. *The effects of high-intensity intermittent exercise training on fat loss and fasting insulin levels of young women.* **E G Trapp, D J Chisholm, J Freund and S H Boutcher.** 2008, Vol. 32, pp. 684 - 691. doi:10.1038/sj.ijo.0803781.

11. *Circulating adiponectin concentration and body composition are altered in response to high-intensity interval training.* **Shing CM, Webb JJ, Driller MW, Williams AD, Fell JW.** 8, s.l. : Journal of Strength and Conditioning, 2013, Vol. 27, pp. 2213 - 2218.

12. *Adiponectin: More Than Just Another Fat Cell Hormone?* **Mandu Chandran, Susan A. Phillips, Theodore Ciaraldi, Robert R. Henry.** 8, s.l. : Diabetes Care, 2003, Vol. 28. 10.2337/diacare.26.8.2442 .

13. **Talisa Emberts, M.S., John P. Porcari, Ph.D., Jeffery Steffen, Ph.D., Scott Doberstein, M.S., and Carl Foster, Ph.D.** Is Tabata All It's Cracked Up To Be? . *ACE.* [Online] 2013. [Cited: 2 5, 2014.] https://www.acefitness.org/prosourcearticle/3497/is-tabata-all-it-s-cracked-up-to-be.

14. *The effects of high-intensity intermittent exercise training on fat loss and fasting insulin levels of young women.* **E G Trapp, D J Chisholm, J Freund and S H Boutcher.** 2008, International Journal of Obesity, Vol. 32, pp. 684 - 691.

Printed in Great Britain
by Amazon